THE BREAST SOURCEBOOK

OTHER BOOKS BY M. SARA ROSENTHAL

The Thyroid Sourcebook, updated edition (1996, Lowell House)
The Gynecological Sourcebook, updated edition (1997, Lowell House)
The Pregnancy Sourcebook, updated edition (1997, Lowell House)
The Fertility Sourcebook (1995, Lowell House)
The Breastfeeding Sourcebook (1995, Lowell House)

THE BREAST SOURCEBOOK

Everything You Need to Know about
Cancer Detection, Treatment, and Prevention

· · · · · · · · ·

M. SARA ROSENTHAL

Foreword by Pamela H. Craig
M.D., F.A.C.S., Ph.D., Surgical Oncologist
The Breast Center

· · · · · ·

Illustrations by Karen Leiser

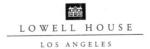

LOWELL HOUSE
LOS ANGELES

CONTEMPORARY BOOKS
CHICAGO

Library of Congress Cataloging-in-Publication Data
Rosenthal, M. Sara
    The breast sourcebook : everything you need to know about breast cancer detec-
tion, treatment, and prevention / M. Sara Rosenthal; foreword by Dawn Holman; illustrations by Karen Leiser.
        p.   cm.
    Includes bibliographical references and index.
    ISBN 1-56565-891-1 (paperback)
    1. Breast—Cancer—Popular works.   I. Title.
RC280.B8R675   1996
616.99'449—dc20

96-43007
CIP

Requests for such permissions should be addressed to:
Lowell House
2020 Avenue of the Stars, Suite 300
Los Angeles, CA 90067

Lowell House books can be purchased at special discounts when ordered in bulk for premiums and special sales. Contact Department TC at the address above.

Publisher: Jack Artenstein
Associate Publisher, Lowell House Adult: Bud Sperry
Director of Publishing Services: Rena Copperman
Managing Editor: Maria Magallanes
Text design: Kate Mueller
Illustrations: Karen Leiser

Manufactured in the United States of America
10 9 8 7 6 5 4 3 2 1

To your mothers, grandmothers, and daughters

CONTENTS

ACKNOWLEDGMENTS

If it weren't for the commitment, hard work, and guidance of the following people, this book would never have been written.

Dawn M. Holman and Joy McDiarmid, producers of the critically acclaimed audiotape support series *Voices in the Night: A Cancer Companion,* offered immediate, unwavering support in this difficult project and put me in touch with their own contacts—something that is rarely done.

Pamela H. Craig, M.D., F.A.C.S., Ph.D., surgical oncologist at The Breast Center in Van Nuys, California, provided encouragement, support, frankness, and a wealth of valuable comments and resources to this work. Gillian Arsenault, M.D., C.C.F.P., I.B.C.L.C., F.R.C.P., Simon Fraser Health Unit, Maple Ridge, British Columbia, my medical adviser on *The Breastfeeding Sourcebook,* walked with me through the sea of epidemiological studies, held my hand, and did not let go. (As luck would have it, Dr. Arsenault had just completed an in-depth report on breast cancer epidemiology when I asked her for her expertise.) Virginia Fraser, M.D., F.R.C.S., Medical Director, Misericordia Hospital Breast Clinic, Winnipeg, Manitoba, made numerous contributions that helped shape this work; Sarah S. Auchincloss, M.D., a psychiatrist at the Memorial Sloan-Kettering Cancer Center, New York City, who specializes in psycho-oncology, took time away from a busy practice and family obligations to contribute her comments and encouragement to this work. Rosalind Benedet, N.P., M.S.N., Clinical Nurse Specialist and Coordinator of the Breast Health Center, California Pacific Medical Center, San Francisco, California, provided me with careful observations and comments, as well as resources on post-mastectomy healing that are difficult to find. Karen Faye, L.P.N., A.F.A.A. (Aerobics and Fitness Association of America) fitness practitioner, provided important comments on prevention and diet. Karen has herself maintained an 80-pound weight loss since 1982. As an oncology nurse with the Well Woman Project at Saints Memorial Hospital, Lowell, Massachussets, a project for wellness education and prevention of women's health problems, Karen is a real pioneer in lifestyle modification. Finally, I owe a great debt to an oncologist known for being a strong patient advocate, who volunteered to read over many more portions of this manuscript than asked and who made necessary, candid comments that helped to reshape my original manuscript into this book; this specialist has asked to remain anonymous.

I'd also like to thank my editorial assistant, journalist Sujata Talreja; the illustrator, Karen Leiser, for her beautiful drawings and attention to detail; and my very patient editor, Maria Magallanes.

Special thanks to Suzanne Pratt, M.D., F.A.C.O.G., who provided so much of the groundwork for this text through her expertise on two of my earlier works.

All the breast cancer survivors interviewed for this book helped to guide me. Your stories, struggles, and important suggestions regarding content were very much appreciated.

In the moral support department my husband, Gary S. Karp, and all the relatives and friends who cheered me on.

FOREWORD

Chances are, if you have this book in hand, you picked it up because you know someone with breast cancer or you have the disease yourself. If it's you who have just been diagnosed with breast cancer, you've probably listened to what your doctor has told you about treatment and prognosis but little has sunk in. You may be in a state of shock, and overwhelmed by fear and panic.

Even after years of being a breast specialist who has counseled many women about surgical treatment options, I had those same feelings myself several years ago when I found out I had breast cancer. I was fortunate because I knew what I had to do and I was already familiar with the medical data. But the sense of big-time foreboding that comes with this diagnosis doesn't spare anyone. To help put a diagnosis in perspective I have always tried to recommend reading materials to patients and friends. Somehow that always seemed a bit too academic, although I know that "taking control" is important and "knowledge is power."

Knowing as much as you can about your disease is especially true now in the era of managed care because your health care provider may not have time to explain all you need to know to make informed decisions about your treatment. In fact, you may still feel a sense of powerlessness and deep awareness that you don't have all that much control over the disease or treatment, but even a little understanding of what is going on helps to quell the panic that can overtake you when you think the worst.

When asked to advise M. Sara Rosenthal on *The Breast Sourcebook,* I asked her why she wanted to do this. She explained that she wanted to present easily readable, yet complete and comprehensive, information, yet not an encyclopedia, nor a bible, but a source that would give all the basics in a language everyone could understand. I think she has achieved her goal and accomplished a Himalayan task magnificently. From clearing the brush from the mammography guidelines controversy to explaining the "language" of treatment options ("tumors have margins like a piece of paper"), Sara clarifies with humor and intelligence ("TNM is not a new cable channel, but a stage classification system currently used.").

While not all women want to hear all the details of their disease and treatment options, most women do want to know more and sometimes may feel their doctor did not give them sufficient information. Most women want to feel they are in a partnership with their physicians as they make treatment decisions and they are entitled to that.

The Breast Sourcebook will help you understand the language we use so you can ask questions about your disease if you want to or explore areas you may not yet understand. Or perhaps you want to use the information for preparing yourself to find physician team members who are better able to communicate with you on whatever level you see fit. This book, for example, has specific sections on dealing with the diagnosis and doctors, what questions you should ask, how to obtain second and third opinions, and how to use a specialist.

There are so many decisions to be made following an initial diagnosis. I too felt overwhelmed at that point and there were questions I felt embarrassed to ask. And as I look back on that time three years ago, I often wonder how anybody gets through it. But you do and you will. As I know from personal experience, even chemotherapy and radiation are tolerable. M. Sara Rosenthal explains the side effects and how to cope with them.

Her book is an excellent starting point for demystifying the more difficult aspects of this disease. She helps to make the vital difference between losing yourself in fear and understanding the problem.

Pamela H. Craig, M.D., Ph.D., F.A.C.S.
The Breast Center, Van Nuys, California
July, 1997

THIS IS NOT THE BOOK
I ORIGINALLY WROTE

When I set out to write a balanced and accurate book about breast health and breast cancer, I knew it was going to be tough, but not nearly as tough as it turned out to be. I discovered that breast cancer is not just a health issue but a minefield of controversy. The first book I wrote was bogged down with the history and politics of breast cancer and dealt with topics ranging from mammography and tamoxifen debates, to research fraud and surefire prevention tips. But that was the *first* book I wrote about breast cancer—a book I had to write, but one you didn't need to read.

The truth is, studies about the causes, risks, and prevention of breast cancer are volatile material. The "good studies" are criticized by one camp, the "bad studies" by another, and the conclusive studies remain inconclusive in so many areas that there are precious few deductions you can make about the disease. There is so much wishful science and politicizing to grapple with, it's very easy to get sucked in and wonder why no one thought of X or Y twenty years ago. I didn't want to do this because I believe that's not my place, especially when there is so much information on breast cancer. My job, as I see it, is to give you the information you need to form your own opinion and make the decisions that are right for you.

Perhaps the most difficult balancing act was figuring out what to do with all the information I had amassed on breast cancer prevention (enough for another complete book). My first instinct was to deal with the subject at the beginning of the book, so readers could benefit right away. But one morning, as I read yet another editorial about yet another controversial risk factor associated with breast cancer that had drawn in angry and panicky letters from across the country, I saw a letter by a woman my age (thirty-three). The letter writer was completely fed up with the never-ending reports that tell women how they could have protected themselves from breast cancer. The woman said that she had developed breast cancer *now* and didn't want to be told any more about how eating more broccoli would have protected her from the disease. So much for the first draft of my prevention chapter, which, funny enough, *did* have a few paragraphs on cruciferous vegetables.

After listening to other breast cancer survivors who shared this view, I started to see the entire subject of breast cancer prevention in a different light. It became clear to me that prevention information is not what most of my readers need or want to read first, because if you are reading this book, you are probably either sweating out a biopsy or have just been diagnosed with the disease—we don't buy books about breast health until we really need the information. As one woman with metastatic disease put it to me, "I want my *daughter* to read your prevention chapter, but *I* need to know more about detection and treatment." Fair enough. I decided that prevention is the future of this disease, not the present, which is why we end with prevention but start with our histories.

So, what else has changed from my first book on breast cancer to *this* one? Well, I think you'll find the information in the book is accurate and unbiased, not an easy thing to do when ten doctors can persuasively argue their individual points of view regarding detection, risk, prevention, and treatment. You'll also find "undoctored" material, which is difficult to get because of the explosive nature of breast cancer issues. I have attempted at every stage to give you accurate and comprehensive information about breast health and breast cancer.

My first chapter will answer the question: Who gets breast cancer, and why? I discuss each risk in detail in alphabetical order, but keep in mind (and I'll remind you when you get there) that 70 percent of the women who develop breast cancer have no known risk factors. This is one reason why so many women are angry and frustrated about the disease, and why so *much* research is going on in so many areas. And since the breast cancer rate is increasing in North America, the push for prevention is extremely strong among both the medical and grassroots community.

Chapter 2 answers the question: *Is* It cancer? This chapter is the one to read if you're worried about a lump you've found, if you have been told you have fibrocystic breast condition, if you are wondering about a breast infection, or if you are unsure about what the next step is. I also discuss the investigation process and mammography guidelines you can follow *in spite* of the conflicting rules and will explain in detail how you do a proper breast self-exam.

Chapter 3, When They Say It's Malignant, sees you through the first few weeks of your diagnosis to your surgery date (if you choose to have surgery). It explains what cancer is, discusses the types and stages of breast cancer, as well as the treatment approaches, and suggests questions you can ask your doctor. If you've had surgery, you can move to Chapter 4, Life after Surgery, which deals with a number of possible treatments you may have after surgery, including radiation therapy, chemotherapy, and hormone therapy. It also discusses postoperative symptoms such as fatigue and lymphedema and the side effects associated with radiation and chemotherapy.

For those women who are considering reconstruction, details about breast reconstruction procedures and types of non-implant and implant procedures are provided in Chapter 5, which also gives you some background on the whole breast implant controversy and discusses alternatives to reconstruction.

Chapter 6, Friends and Lovers, prepares you for the changes breast cancer may make in your sexual relationships and suggests ways to communicate with your sex partner and repair your love life. The chapter also discusses fertility and pregnancy issues.

Chapter 7 tells you All about Complementary Medicine, the alternative, non-Western approaches to cancer. The pros and cons of each approach are discussed.

Chapter 8, The Second Time Around, is the place to go for information about recurrence or metastatic disease. Chapter 9 discusses Palliative Care in detail, as well as some issues involved in end-stage breast cancer.

Chapter 10 answers the question: What about Prevention? It tells you how you can be proactive about breast cancer and what you can realistically do to make your body as healthy as possible. It does not give you a recipe for preventing breast cancer, however, since no such recipe exists. And believe me, I looked. Finally, I've provided a glossary to help you with various terms in the book.

Don't forget to check the back of the book for resources: lists of breast cancer organizations and instructions on how to access breast cancer information on-line.

Now, here's what I'd like *you* to do. Write to me care of the publisher or e-mail me at MSara2@aol.com if there's information you'd like that's not in here. Chances are I have the information, and if I don't, I'll get it for you. If you include a self-addressed stamped envelope, fax number, or e-mail address, I'll be glad to send it out to you. Little by little, we'll make this book the best sourcebook about breast health and breast cancer. I think this book is a good start, and I'm proud to have my name on it.

CHAPTER 1

WHO GETS BREAST CANCER, AND WHY?

In the United States one woman dies from breast cancer every twelve minutes. The often quoted one-in-eight figure reflects a *lifetime risk* assuming that you live to be ninety-five. In 1940, this lifetime risk was only one in twenty; between 1973 and 1988, it rose by 25 percent.

Surveys show that women vastly underestimate their risk of dying of a heart attack, while they overestimate their chances of dying of breast cancer. About six times as many women die of a heart attack than of breast cancer.

This chapter aims to answer the question, "who gets breast cancer, and why?" For the most part, the answer is "we really don't know," but by the end of this chapter, you'll have a much better understanding of how breast cancer risk is calculated and interpreted. For women who do not have a family history of breast cancer, it seems that how you live, where you live and work, what you eat, and what you breathe have more to do with your breast cancer risk than your genes. In other words, there is considerable (although circumstantial) evidence that breast cancer risk may vary considerably with environment and lifestyle. In order to understand breast cancer risk, it's important to forget most of what you've heard or read about risk in the past. That's because known risk factors, discussed in this chapter, account for less than 30 percent of all breast cancers.

Finally, I'll discuss an emerging science in the breast cancer industry: risk counseling. Because the information about risk is so confusing and conflicting, many women don't know what to believe. Risk counseling is something you may want to consider if your fear of the disease is interfering with your quality of life. I hope you'll take comfort in the fact that most women overestimate their risk by at least four times.

REVIEWING THE KNOWN RISK FACTORS

What should you understand when you're told you're at risk for breast cancer or any other disease? A few things, depending on the adjective that precedes the word *risk*.

When trying to understand risk factors, having a degree in actuarial science really helps. A risk that is quoted can be either an estimate or based on the experiences of a real group of people, but it is always an average of the experience of that group. So, an estimate of risk is a guess based on information that may include breast cancer mortalities in a given area or age group or mortalities of women who share your medical history. Risk is *not* based on you personally, but on estimates based on the past experience of women like you or, at least, who are like you in terms of the characteristics we know. It's like betting in a horse race. You look at the ages of the horses, their histories, the breeding, the jockeys, and where the race is being run to come up with odds. When you read in this book, for example, that one in eight women over a lifetime will get breast cancer, this is an average risk. The problem with an average risk is that it tends to underestimate risk in some women and overestimate risk in others. In short, any estimate of risk is risk prediction based on information from the past.

So how exactly does one estimate risk? Well, epidemiologists start by watching groups of people. They notice that some people get breast cancer and some don't. They look at the cases occurring per year (annual number of cases), or cases per 10,000 women per year (annual incidence rate), or cases per 10,000 women at each age (age-specific incidence rate), or the number of cases that occur in 10,000 women from birth to age fifty (premenopausal incidence rate). All these people are counted up, and epidemiologists will simply describe what they've seen. Then they look to the future and try to predict risk based on what they've seen and counted. So, let's say you read that one in two hundred women will get breast cancer by age forty-five. That means that from the day you were born, your chance of getting breast cancer is one in two hundred. But if you're already forty-four and do not have breast cancer, your risk of getting breast cancer by next year is much less than one in two hundred because you've made it this far already.

There is a world of difference between absolute, cumulative, relative, and attributable risk. Absolute risk is counted in number of cancer cases occurring within a group of people. When you hear, for example, that fifty out of a hundred thousand women died last year of breast cancer, absolute risk is being discussed. The official definition of absolute risk is the "observed or calculated probability of an event in a population under study." Here, population could be hypothetical or real, it's just not compared to any *other* population.

Cumulative risk is added-up risk. It is the risk per unit of time added up over X units of time, such as a lifetime or a given time frame a study ran. Then there's relative risk, which is based on a comparison of two populations. When I discuss the theory that women who eat large amounts of fat are at greater risk for breast cancer than women who have low-fat diets, I'm discussing relative risk. It directly compares a population of women who have one type of risk factor (eating a high-fat diet, for example) to a population of women who have a different risk factor (eating a low-fat diet), that is, it compares risk in situation A with risk in situation B (which is usually a standard or constant, such as no risk factor).

Of course, women who eat large amounts of fat can alter their diets, and women who smoke can quit smoking. When you speak of risk that can be reduced, prevented, or altered through behavior (like quitting smoking or dieting) or passing legislation to make, say, tobacco illegal, you're now talking about modifiable risk because it is under voluntary control. This is different from a risk marker such as family history, which cannot be modified. Finally comes attributable risk, which refers to a component of one's risk attributable to either a modifiable risk factor, such as diet, or a risk marker, such as family history.

Breast cancer is not like lung cancer. We know that at least 70 percent of people who get lung cancer are smokers and, conversely, that smokers have a far higher risk of getting lung cancer than nonsmokers. Not only that, but the relationship between smoking and getting lung cancer is the same through different time periods and cultures and continents. The more you smoke and the longer you smoke, the higher your risk, and when you stop, your risk drops. Therefore, you can confidently say that smoking causes lung cancer, a cancer which kills more women each year than any other cancer. You can't pinpoint one main cause of breast cancer. All you can do is count up the women who are diagnosed with the disease, compare their lifestyles and family histories to the women without breast cancer, and analyze the effects of each factor.

What most of us have been bombarded with since the 1970s are reports of *known* risk factors such as age, family history, and diet. It's important to note that only about 30 percent of all breast cancers can be explained by known risk factors. For younger women (ages thirty to fifty-four), these risk factors account for an even lower percentage of risk of just 20 percent. It's also important to understand that many of the known risks are conflicting and often controversial. While one study suggests that this or that increases your risk, another study may suggest the contrary.

Statistics are very tricky. For example, if the probability is less than one in twenty of something being found *by chance*, it is statistically significant. Therefore, even if a certain characteristic, such as eye color, has absolutely no effect on breast cancer, for every twenty studies that conclude eye color results in no difference between cases of women with breast cancer and women without breast cancer, one study will show a significant departure from that conclusion. So when a report is "statistically significant," remember that this finding was made purely by chance. Though the media may be going wild, the next nineteen studies won't show anything, and those nineteen studies won't get the same coverage the first study got. (If the next nineteen studies showed the same difference, however, then we could be more sure about the relationship between the characteristic studied and breast cancer, but this still doesn't mean that the characteristic causes breast cancer.)

The bottom line is, don't jump to conclusions when you hear breaking news about a new risk. It's also important to understand that no one, single, personal risk factor such as age or diet can be interpreted as the one and only cause of breast cancer. There are many lifestyle changes you can make to significantly lower your risks. In addition, understanding the impact of the environment on breast cancer will help you put these risks in perspective. Since the list of known risk factors are long, I've decided to discuss all of them, be they gospel or controversy. One factor I don't discuss is the left-handed trait, which, curiously, has been found to reduce risk in the two out of the three studies that investigated it.

Another final distinction I need to make before you go through this list on known risk factors is the difference between *association* and *causation*. Almost everything discussed in this chapter is association *not* causation. When you see a sentence like, "women with breast cancer were found to eat more fat than women without breast cancer," this means association. It does *not* mean that dietary fat causes breast cancer. Causation is when you see the sentence "smoking causes lung cancer."

The following list is arranged alphabetically to make it easier for you to access information you may want right now.

AGE

The risk of breast cancer is largely age-related. It's rare to see breast cancer under age 30, less common to see it between the ages of 30 and 40, and most common in developed nations after menopause (or after age 50). North American statistics from 1984 to 1988 show the following pattern of breast cancer incidence among age groups:

- In women 20 to 24: 0.9 per 100,000 women
- In women 30 to 34: 187.4 per 100,000 women
- In women 50 to 54: 220 per 100,000 women
- In women 65 to 69: 390.7 per 100,000 women
- In women 75 to 79: 461.4 per 100,000 women

So again, the one-in-eight figure refers to your cumulative risk over a lifetime, assuming that you live to age 95.

You can also look at your cumulative risk (risk from birth to a given age)

Table 1.1

YOUR RISK OF GETTING BREAST CANCER

By age 25	• • •	one in 19,608
By age 30	• • •	one in 2,525
By age 35	• • •	one in 622
By age 40	• • •	one in 217
By age 45	• • •	one in 93
By age 50	• • •	one in 50
By age 55	• • •	one in 33
By age 60	• • •	one in 24
By age 65	• • •	one in 17
By age 70	• • •	one in 14
By age 75	• • •	one in 11
By age 80	• • •	one in 10
By age 85	• • •	one in 9
Ever	• • •	one in 8

Source: National Cancer Institute

when it's broken down into five-year intervals (using American statistics). But, the older you get, the less you need to worry about your cumulative risk. You've "been there, done that," and did not get breast cancer. So a 75-year-old woman without breast cancer who plans to live to age 100 has a one-in-eleven to one-in-eight risk of getting breast cancer over the course of the rest of her life.

BAD HABITS

Any lifestyle indulgence that has proven to be a risk factor for something you don't want to happen to you is, for the purposes of this chapter, a bad habit. If you smoke, drink an excessive amount of alcohol, or abuse illegal drugs, your risk of getting some diseases is higher than people who don't do these things.

Alcohol and cigarettes have been linked to a variety of cancers; breast cancer is no exception. A 1994 survey conducted by the American Cancer Society suggested that smokers were 25 percent more likely than nonsmokers or ex-smokers to die of breast cancer. This is different than saying "smoking causes breast cancer," however. It might be saying, "nonsmokers have a better chance of avoiding breast cancer than smokers." It might also mean that smokers who get breast cancer are more likely to die of it. However, smoking does conclusively cause lung cancer.

As for alcohol, a 1993 National Institutes of Health study found that two alcoholic drinks per day could raise your estrogen levels enough to increase your risk of breast cancer by 40 to 100 percent over women who do not drink at all. In this study, thirty-four women had their blood levels checked mid-cycle and were found to have a 31.9 percent increase in estrogen over women who were not drinking. Of course, it's also been shown that between one to two glasses of wine per day for men and one to three alcoholic beverages per week for women may lower the risk of heart disease. The alcohol raises your HDL (high density lipid fraction, the good cholesterol) and reduces the deposits of cholesterol in the arterial walls.

As for illegal drugs, such as cocaine, the risks of an overdose or developing other health problems, such as strokes or AIDS from intravenous drug use, is the main concern.

BRAS

In his book *Dressed to Kill: The Link between Breast Cancer and Bras,* medical anthropologist Sydney Ross Singer raises the question of whether bras cause breast cancer. He compared women in five United States cities who wore bras with those who didn't. He concluded that women who wore bras had a higher breast cancer risk. Based on interviews with 4,700 women, Singer and his coauthor claim that bras constrict the lymph system preventing it from draining and flushing out toxins. The buildup of toxins in breast tissue, according to Singer, triggers lumps, bumps, and cancer. Medical doctors say this is pure nonsense, pointing out that if this were true most breast cancers would not occur in breasts where the bras restrict the least! According to Singer, wearing a bra twenty-four hours a day increases a woman's risk 125-fold, but removing it for two weeks cures fibrocystic breast condition, which is not a diagnosis of breast cancer, as discussed in Chapter 2. According to medical doctors, Singer's hypothesis is a complete fallacy because there are many women who do not wear bras and still have fibrocystic breast condition. Doctors call Singer's study bad science or "junk" science because he has not factored out the influence of other significant risk factors, such as diet. One doctor wrote to me that "[Singer's] study is just awful. You could use his methods to prove anything you want."

But Singer may have stumbled across a factor that may have some bearing on breast cancer, namely the breast being held too close to body temperature. Males with undescended testicles have been found to have a higher incidence of testicular cancer. Some medical texts also note that girls who wear tight bras can develop hyperprolactinemia, a condition in which there's too much prolactin in your system.

Singer also points out the notion that braless cultures in Africa or Asia have lower rates of breast cancer, while African- and Asian-American women who wear bras have higher rates of breast cancer. Keep in mind though that the diet in these braless cultures are lower in fat and often high in fish and sea vegetables and that women have more children, have their first children at an *earlier* age, and breastfeed longer. In addition, North America is more industrialized, and where there's industry, there are higher rates of breast cancer, as well as cultural differences such as fewer children, later first children, less breastfeeding, and higher longevity rates. So don't burn your bra just yet, but you can certainly go braless if you like. Massaging your breasts daily apparently helps get the blood flowing properly. Going braless increases the progression of "Cooper's droop," in which the supporting ligaments of the breasts, called Cooper's ligaments, stretch under the influence of gravity. This stretching is inevitable as we age, but lessened when a bra is worn for external support.

In fact, some theories hold that nipple stimulation of any sort, be it sex play or breastfeeding, may reduce breast cancer risk by clearing free radicals and/or raising oxytocin and lowering prolactin (hormones that control milk production). I'll keep you posted in future editions about this phenomenon.

DEMOGRAPHICS

Rates of breast cancer depend largely on where one lives. Industrialized countries have much higher breast cancer rates than underdeveloped countries. The World Health Organization (WHO) estimates that the industrial average (meaning cumulative, or lifetime, average) hovers at roughly one in eleven in industrialized countries.

A 1986 survey found that the countries with the highest *pre*menopausal breast cancer rates were Australia and New Zealand, while North America had the highest *post*menopausal breast cancer rate. Japan's lifetime rate was the lowest in the industrialized world, which was five times less than the industrial average. Eleven Japanese women out of 100,000 will develop breast cancer in their lifetimes, compared to 50 out of 100,000 women in New Zealand, and 46 out of 100,000 women in Germany.

An interesting demographic anomaly showed up recently in Newton, Massachusetts, where breast cancer rates were 23 percent higher than the state average. The higher rates were found among more affluent women and Jewish women. Roughly 1 in 40 Jewish women carry genes that cause inherited breast cancer (see further on). Affluent women (of all races) are also more likely to seek out breast screening and perform self exams, which may account for a higher incidence. They're also more likely to delay childbirth, drive cars (less exercise), and perhaps consume higher fat diets.

All over the map

The key word when it comes to calculating global risk is *region*. Rates of breast cancer can be dramatically different between regions, although we just don't know why. For instance, the breast cancer rate in Geneva is double that in Spain, even though they are not that far apart geographically. In San Francisco, the rate is double that in Newfoundland, proving that breast cancer in North America can vary from coast to coast.

Even more interesting, a 1992 *New England Journal of Medicine* article concluded that people migrating from regions with low rates of breast cancer increased their risk when migrating to a country with higher incidences of breast cancer. This suggests that breast cancer is largely affected by environmental factors, which could include lifestyle, culture, diet, water, and air quality.

The risk of breast cancer in North America is also about 30 percent higher in urban communities than in rural ones and, as a result, is higher in black communities than in white. Five-year survival rates (1980-1990) were 82 percent for Caucasian women and 66 percent for black women. Yet incidence rates for postmenopausal breast cancer are highest among Caucasian women, followed by African-, Hispanic-, and Asian- North American women. Premenopausal breast cancer (i.e. breast cancer under age 45), is highest in African-North American women. Women in a higher socioeconomic class, regardless of race have a higher incidence of breast cancer as well because of access to screening and health care delivery—the same reason why survival rates are lower in black women.

Global statistics also vary when it comes to mortality and incidence rates. Currently, women in the United Kingdom are more likely to die of breast cancer each year than in any other country; breast cancer is the single most common cause of deaths for British women between the ages thirty-five and fifty-four. But the incidence of getting breast cancer is even higher in North America. In fact, the one-in-eight lifetime risk is expected to be revised to one in seven by the year 2000.

Even in Japan, where the breast cancer rate is one of the lowest of the industrialized world, the incidence of the disease is still increasing. For example, Osaka witnessed in the thirty to seventy-four age group, an increase from an annual incidence rate of about 27 in 100,000 women in 1970, to about 49 in 100,000 women in 1985.

To grasp just how much breast cancer has risen in the last decade, it's important to remember that the incidence of the disease remained fairly stable from 1940 to 1980, rising at about 1 percent each year. However, between 1980 and 1985, the rate of breast cancer increased by 21 percent in the United States (15 percent in Canada), and the incidence rate has been skyrocketing ever since, making breast cancer truly epidemic. When you add everything up, the rate of breast cancer rose 34 percent among white women and 47 percent among black women between 1973 and 1992. By the year 2000, the annual mortality rate from breast cancer in the developed world is expected to top one million. A logical question at this point might be: What caused such a dramatic increase to take place? It's only natural to wonder whether a dramatic cause can be linked to these statistics. There are many theories. For example, see pages 30–36 for more information on how industry may play a role in environmental disruption and cancer risk.

DIET

Diet plays an enormous role in our health, as many studies tracking the role of diet have concluded. In terms of breast cancer, because it has been suggested that higher levels of estrogen may be associated with a higher risk of breast cancer, it's important to be moderate in our intake of certain foods which increase the estrogen levels in our body. These include:

- *Fat.* Our fat cells make estrogen. The more fat we eat, the bigger our fat cells get and the more estrogen they make.
- *Meat.* Even organically raised meat such as free-range chicken can still be exposed to pesticides (which may contain estrogenic mimics from the vegetation they ingest and can wind up inside our own bodies, contributing to an estrogen overload. Meat is also higher in fat. (But as omnivores, our bodies are meant to eat a certain amount of meat and other animal products, which are good sources of amino acids, iron, vitamin B_{12}, and zinc.)
- *Other animal products, such as eggs, milk, and milk products.*
- *Fish.* If the fish you eat is from contaminated waters, you may be ingesting mercury or PCBs, which get stored in your fat. Seafood containing mercury may not cause as many symptoms because it's high in selenium, which apparently counteracts the immediate toxic effects of mercury poisoning. Otherwise, fish that is contaminant-free is quite healthy.

Numerous studies suggest that women who eat less fat and meat and more fruits, fiber, and vegetables may be less at risk for breast cancer. The evidence comes from cross-cultural comparisons where other factors besides diet may be at work. While a healthy, low-fat diet is certainly good and will definitely reduce your risk of heart disease and stroke (more women die from heart disease than from any other illness), it isn't the secret to breast cancer prevention. However it holds a lot of promise. I've devoted a significant amount of space to the subject of diet in Chapter 10, pages 250–264.

It's also worth noting that sea vegetables, which are high in soluble iodines, have been shown in animal studies and human cross-cultural studies to have some protective effect against breast cancer.

ENVIRONMENTAL FACTORS

Environmental factors are probably significant when assessing risk of breast cancer. While radiation exposure from modern-day low-dose diagnostic X rays is not considered a concern by the medical establishment, high-dose radiation exposure is. (See below for examples of high-dose radiation.) For example, if your breasts were exposed to high-dose radiation, this can increase your risk of breast cancer—especially if you were exposed around the time of your first menstrual period to a high-dose X ray or radiation emitted during a nuclear explosion or accident.

For the record, women living near areas with high levels of radioactive fallout have higher incidence of a variety of cancers—including breast cancer. Female survivors of Hiroshima and Nagasaki who were extensively followed showed a dramatic increase in breast cancer rates, particularly with women in their teens and twenties. The highest number of breast cancer cases were seen in women who were exposed to fallout when they were less than ten years of age. Women who were older at exposure did not seem to be vulnerable to this effect. Breasts may become more resistant to radiation as they mature.

Similar studies have backed up this early radiation exposure risk. In North America, women checked for tuberculosis as children with fluoroscopy (high-dose X rays taken as a child breathed in) during the 1930s and 1940s were found to have higher rates of breast cancer. A Rochester study found that women treated with radiation for mastitis (bacterial breast infection) from the 1920s to 1960s also had higher rates of breast cancer. The same was true for women treated as children with radiation for acne, for enlarged thymus glands (as infants), and anyone subjected to the equivalent of one X ray per week for two years during childhood (sometimes done for scoliosis). Radiation was also widely used to determine fetal positions in prenatal care (during the 1930s and 1940s, known as pelvimetry, which exposed the fetal breast tissue to radiation), and was used to treat asthma, pneumonia, whooping cough, and even hyperthyroidism (today, radioactive iodine is used, which is not linked to breast cancer). Let's not forget the radiation used to treat congenital heart problems, as well as those standard TB exams most employers demanded between 1920 and 1960. Radiation was also widely used by chiropractors to determine spinal column alignment, and shoe retailers, who used high dose x-rays on the feet to find out shoe size.

John W. Gofman, M.D., Ph.D., in his book *Preventing Breast Cancer: The Story of a Major, Proven, Preventable Cause of This Disease* (1995), concludes that about three-fourths of breast cancer cases are largely due to past medical-related radiation. In other words, according to Gofman, women who received radiation as children or young women may be able to link their breast cancers to that period in their life. He also suggests that much of the radiation therapy between the 1920s and 1960s was probably poorly documented (i.e. much more was done than we think). Gofman states that 75 percent of the women who have recently had breast cancer or are currently diagnosed would probably never have developed it if medicine had never used irradiation. Gofman also states that there is no safe level of radiation; even low-dose radiation can cause cancer (but at much lower rates than high-dose radiation). Some studies have found the increase in breast cancer risk is directly proportional to the radiation dose.

Electromagnetic fields

Researchers are still trying to see whether electromagnetic fields (for example, areas near power lines) can predispose people who live or people who work near them to higher rates of cancer. This hasn't yet been proven, but if there is an association, it's quite small.

Electric blankets are one source of electromagnetic fields, and one theory suggests cancer risk increases with how much one uses these blankets. Those who use electric blankets continuously through the night may be at a somewhat higher risk than those who use it daily but not through the night; while those who use it daily may be at higher risk than those who never use it. This risk did not increase with the number of years electric blankets were used, suggesting that the electromagnetic fields associated with electric blankets aren't related to triggering breast cancer so much with as stimulating growth of a cancer already present.

Similarly, three studies found that breast cancer risk in men increased by two times with occupational exposure to electromagnetic fields. (Occupational exposure to electromagnetic fields involves much stronger fields.)

ESTROGEN

High levels of estrogen seem to be associated with increased risk of breast cancer. But the estrogen issue is complicated, since there are times in a woman's life when estrogen levels are high (such as during pregnancy or during certain times in your cycle). Fat cells also make small amounts of estrogen, but this isn't a concern until after menopause, when the ovaries stop making estrogen. Sources of extra estrogen include:

- *Exposure to DES (diethylstilbestrol).* DES is a drug that was administered to pregnant women from the 1940s to the 1970s with the aim of preventing miscarriage. DES daughters are at risk for a variety of reproductive cancers, mainly vaginal and cervical but also including breast cancer. For more information, contact The DES Cancer Network at (510) 465-4011.
- *High-dose birth control pills.* It's no longer necessary for most women to be on high-dose birth control unless your cycles need to be controlled for some reason. Re-visit your pill prescription and find out if it is a low-dose pill. See the separate section on oral contraceptives on page 26.
- *Low-dose birth control pills.* Again, see the separate section on contraception.
- *Hormone replacement therapy.* (See the following section below.)
- *Dietary fat.* (See diet section above and the diet section in Chapter 10.) Dietary fat is not an external source of estrogen, but may contribute to your fat cells' production of estrogen if the fat you eat makes you fat.
- *Environmental estrogens.* (See the section on pages 32–38.)
- *Hormone-fed produce.* (See diet section above, and the diet section in Chapter 10.)

Keep in mind, though, that estrogen levels are difficult to measure in any meaningful way. Estrogen levels can vary with the time of day, menstrual cycle, pregnancy, and lactation. Studies which base their conclusions on a single measurement of estrogen in women may result in confusing or contradictory results. The reading will be true for each woman at the time it was taken, but whether a one-shot reading can be taken as an indicator of overall estrogen exposure is questionable.

EXERCISE

Like diet, exercise also plays a huge role in health. The more we exercise, the more fat we burn, the more oxygen is carried to our muscles, and the better our bodies work. On average, women who do four hours of exercise per week may reduce their risks of premenopausal breast cancer by as much as 58 percent. Lean women, women under 45, and women who exercise regularly three to five times a week, are among those who will witness the greatest risk reduction from exercise. Women with no children lower their risks by 27 percent, while women with children lower their risks by as much as 72 percent. But again, exercise is only *associated* with lower breast cancer risk. We don't know what *other* factors are at work. Are both diet and exercise and some other unknown factor associated with breast cancer risk? Are women who are predisposed to breast cancer less inclined to exercise anyway? We just don't know. What we do know is that strenuous exercise decreases ovarian function and hence estrogen levels are lowered. In addition, by lowering body fat, you're lowering estrogen levels in fat stores as well as reducing insulin resistance, which may also play a role in breast cancer. And women who begin exercising in their teen years may either delay the onset of their periods while reducing the number of lifetime menstrual cycles. In athletes, for example, periods may stop altogether (called amennorhea), which does lower breast cancer risk but also results in thin, brittle bones. What we also know is that people who exercise regularly also tend to eat better. Compared to sedentary women, women who exercise regularly also have higher levels of education, income, and smoke and drink less. All of these factors need to be weighed as well.

The younger you begin regular exercise, the more you may be protected from breast cancer. Even so, women who don't get started until later in life are still more protected than women who are sedentary.

FAMILY HISTORY

The fact that some families are predisposed to cancer was first recorded by the Romans in 100 A.D. Many cancers run in families, particularly breast, ovarian, and colon cancers, among others. That's why research into specific cancer genes is an important step in identifying women at risk. First-degree relatives (parents, siblings, and children) are the ones who are considered in determining whether or not you have a strong family history of breast cancer. In order for you to qualify as having a strong family history of breast cancer, either your mother or sister, or, on rare occasions, your daughter would have to have been diagnosed with breast cancer. The younger they were at the time of diagnosis, the more at risk you are. Grandmothers, great aunts, and paternal relatives are not as crucial in determining family histories. However, if breast cancer was diagnosed in your maternal aunt (your mother's sister), there is a greater likelihood that breast cancer runs in the family. Familial breast cancer, however, accounts for only 5 to 10 percent of all breast cancers. One study also found that daughters of men with prostate cancer were at a higher risk of developing breast cancer.

What about genes?

Since about 1940, researchers have known that cancer is caused by mutating cells. Mutation used to be attributed to aging cells in aging bodies, but we now realize that there are genes that control mutation. And, some genes have more control over mutation than others. A phenomenon called an oncogene is a dormant gene that absorbs various external "hits" until it switches "on," and tells our cells to mutate. Some of us may never have any of our oncogenes turn on, but many of us will. So the question is: Are there specific genes that make some of us more susceptible to a carcinogen, such as tobacco or pesticides? A recent study identified a mutated gene called TSG101, which is found in the majority of breast cancers. It's thought that TSG101 may act as a tumor suppresser gene which mutates, triggering precancerous cells to "grow up" into real cancer. Tests showed that seven out of fifteen breast cancer patients had mutated or missing TSG101.

As for specific cancer mutations present during reproduction, only a small number of cancers have been shown to be genetically inherited in this way. Most research is trying to pin down what switches on some oncogenes and not others.

How carcinogens work

According to what's called the two-stage carcinogenesis theory, a healthy cell is genetically damaged by substances called initiators. A damaged cell will be harmless so long as it doesn't reproduce before the hit is repaired; most hits are repaired. The human body is quite efficient at repairing itself. But people who inherit a defective repair mechanism will age more rapidly and be more susceptible to more cancer.

Even after initiation has occurred, the process of cell damage can still be reversible. That's where substances called *inhibitors* act in a number of ways. They can act like brakes, discouraging cells from transforming into cancerous cells by either preventing the absorption of too much carcinogen or by slowing down the metabolism of the substance. Inhibitors can also reduce the number of cells at risk and enhance DNA repair. Many foods and vitamins have been identified as possible inhibitors (discussed further in Chapter 10).

However, if a "hit" isn't repaired, substances called *promoters* encourage these damaged cells to grow and divide and/or alter the body's immune mechanism in some way. The same substance or exposure can act both as an initiator and a promoter, such as ionizing radiation. Some chemicals and some viruses can act as initiators as well. It can take decades for a cancer to develop after exposure to an initiator, but the period between exposure to promoters and cancer development tends to be shorter. In other words, the lag time between a promoter and cancer is shorter than the lag time between an initiator and cancer.

The breast cancer gene

We have recently discovered that several inherited abnormal genes can cause susceptibility to certain cancers, including BRCA1, BRCA2, and BRCA3. BRCA-2 is mutated in 45 percent of all familial breast cancer cases, while BRCA-1 is linked to both breast and ovarian cancer. Researchers seem to think that both of these genes interact with a third gene, known as Rad51. Another mutated gene called ataxia telangiectasia (ATM) is believed to raise a woman's risk of getting breast cancer by five times, but more studies (obviously!) need to be done. The most well-known breast cancer gene is BRCA1, and women who have this gene are more susceptible to breast cancer than those who don't. It is possible to be screened for this gene, but doing mass screenings is not very useful because this gene accounts for only 4 percent of all breast cancers. It is also found in women who don't get breast cancer and in those who come from low-risk families, although we don't know what finding BRCA1 in a woman without a high-risk family means (if it means anything at all). So, screening everyone would probably scare people for no good reason. A Utah study found that when healthy women were told they had a breast cancer gene, they experienced post-traumatic stress levels almost as high as actual cancer patients. There are probably many other genes—good and bad—that have a role in the development of breast cancer; researchers just haven't discovered them yet. Another problem with screening is that there is no way to tell a woman without the BRCA1 gene that she's *not* at risk for breast cancer since there are so many other factors involved. At this point, it would be better to spend research money on something that conclusively saves lives.

It is estimated that one in three hundred women carry BRCA1 and that it's responsible for 5 percent of all breast cancer cases. In women under 30, however, the BRCA1 gene is implicated in 25 percent of cases. In Ashkenazi Jewish women (Jews of Eastern European descent), BRCA1 and BRCA2, respectively, occur in about 1 percent of that population. Overall, roughly 1 in 40 Ashkenazi Jewish women will test positive for either the BRCA1 or BRCA2 gene.

What if you have the BRCA1 gene?
If you are both BRCA1-positive and from a high-risk family, it's estimated that there's an 85 percent chance that you may develop breast cancer before age eighty, although about 50 percent of women who fall into this group will develop the disease before they are fifty. It has also been found that women who are BRCA1-positive and come from high-risk families typically have half of all female members affected with breast cancer. However, if you have BRCA1 and come from a low-risk family, nobody knows for sure what this means, if it means anything at all.

The BRCA1 is a dominant gene, but behaves like a recessive gene in our bodies. It kicks into action only when its normal partner gene (which may be a tumor suppresser gene) is either lost or becomes inactive.

About genetic testing

In order to determine whether the cancer in your family is genetic, it is recommended that you and your family go for genetic counseling. This is important because predictive genetic testing is a relatively new field with few guidelines for testing, so practitioners have little experience. Genetic counselors document your family history to check if you say "yes" to any of the following statements:

1. Cancers have occurred in three or more of your family members.
2. Cancers have occurred before age forty in your family members.
3. One or more people in your family have developed more than one cancer (for example, separate cancers in each breast or ovarian cancer).
4. Members of your family have closely related cancers (for example, breast, ovary, colon, endometrial, and uterus —these cancers are all hormone related). Keep in mind that hormone replacement therapy, where both estrogen and progestin are used after menopause, almost completely prevents endometrial cancer.

The implications of a positive or negative family history need to be considered carefully. Again, neither is a guarantee of cancer or no cancer in your lifetime. If necessary, a genetic counselor will recommend screening methods such as screening mammogram or colonoscopy. Some experts recommend beginning mammograms at age twenty-five if you're considered at high risk for breast cancer and at age twenty if family members develop breast cancer in their thirties. Not all experts agree with these recommendations, however.

More controversy surrounds other recommendations to women with a high-risk family who have the BRCA1 gene. Recommendations may involve a bilateral mastectomy, oophorectomy (removal of the ovaries), and/or taking tamoxifen as prevention therapy. The pros and cons of each recommendation must be thoroughly discussed with more than one cancer expert. All these prevention measures are discussed thoroughly in Chapter 10.

FERTILITY DRUGS

Fertility drugs, such as clomiphene citrate, cause the ovaries to make many more follicles per month than they normally would. The debate is whether a super-ovulated ovary, and megahits of estrogen in the body, predisposes a woman to ovarian cancer. If the answer is yes then, in theory, it should also predispose you to breast cancer. So here's the deal: If you get pregnant on fertility drugs, these drugs do not increase your risk of either cancer. If you don't get pregnant, your risk is slightly increased for ovarian cancer. The impact on breast cancer is still unknown.

HAIR DYE

The latest conclusion is that hair dye does *not* increase your risk of breast cancer. Past studies have linked hair dye to cancer, particularly black hair dyes designed to cover gray. One study found that women using permanent black dye for more than twenty years increased their risk of rare cancers, such as non-Hodgkin's lymphoma (the cancer that took Jacqueline Kennedy Onassis's life) and melanoma by about four times. A Nebraska study found that hair dye may account for as much as 20 percent of all non-Hodgkin's lymphoma deaths in women. This study also indicated a link between ovarian cancer and breast cancer, but several critics have argued that this study was flawed. So go ahead and dye your hair if you like. If you're uneasy, you can simply switch to an organic or vegetable-based dye.

HORMONE REPLACEMENT THERAPY

It's still unclear whether hormone replacement therapy (HRT) increases your risk of breast cancer, but there is actually more consensus in the medical research community over this issue than many others. That's because the incidence of breast cancer in Western nations dramatically rises after menopause—whether you're on HRT or not. So it's not clear whether HRT *really* contributes to this increase. The current thinking seems to be that if you're on HRT, there is a slight increased risk of developing breast cancer, *but* if you do develop it, it's more likely to be the more treatable breast cancer that is estrogen-receptor positive, which may explain why HRT decreases your risk of dying from breast cancer. HRT has been shown to reduce the risk of dying from breast cancer by 16 percent.

If you add up all the data, you may want to re-think HRT if your risk of breast cancer is high (due to family history, for example), or if the risk of breast cancer significantly outweighs your risk of heart disease. For the record, heart disease kills far more women than breast cancer, and HRT can definitely lower your cholesterol levels, lower your risk of heart disease, and lower your risk of dying from heart disease. Furthermore, if you are at greater risk for osteoporosis, HRT stops bone loss (all women are at risk but those who exercise or have heavier bones will not develop it as quickly). In fact, HRT can even increase bone mass if started in the first few years after menopause. Remember hip and spinal fractures can be very debilitating (often life-threatening) and can truly affect quality of life.

If you're on HRT and are diagnosed with breast cancer . . .

A recent 1995 study in Ottawa, Ontario, found that women on HRT had more difficulty battling breast cancer once it was diagnosed. This led to a scare in Canada that turned out to be unnecessary. Doctors will simply take you off hormone replacement therapy if breast cancer is diagnosed, completely eliminating the problem and restoring your survival rate to that of the general population. That said, many medical papers suggest that women undergoing breast cancer treatment can still be on HRT; HRT is not necessarily contraindicated in all women who have had breast cancer.

MENSTRUAL HISTORY

Your menstrual history can also apparently affect your risk of breast cancer, but many experts have conflicting opinions as to how important a role it plays. For example, one factor is what experts call early menarche. Menarche refers to your first period; early menarche means that you got your first period prior to age twelve. This apparently trivial detail also suggests that you've been producing estrogen longer than the average woman, which is why this is considered.

Menarche levels can vary enormously. The average age of menarche is 12.8 years old in the United States but 17 years in China, which is why some researchers say this may help to explain why breast cancer occurrence in China is one-third that of the United States And even within China, provinces with later menarche tend to have lower rates of breast cancer.

Another factor is cycle length. If your periods are either further apart or closer together than average, your breast cancer risk increases by some estimates as high as 50 percent. (An average cycle is anywhere from twenty-six to twenty-nine days.) Shorter or longer cycles indicate a hormonal imbalance at work, which *may* contribute to an increased breast cancer risk. Shorter cycles also indicate that you're spending more time in a high-estrogen portion of your cycle.

Keep in mind that in the last century, women became pregnant almost as soon as they got their first periods. They would simply continue getting pregnant until they reached menopause or dropped dead in their mid-30s due to terrible living conditions or childbirth. Women would average about six children, breastfeed for extended time frames (breastfeeding delays ovulation, which is why it protects you from breast and ovarian cancers), and ultimately, not have more than about 20 periods in a lifetime! Women today have 300-400 periods in a lifetime, exposing the breasts to record levels of estrogen due to the sheer number of cycles.

ORAL CONTRACEPTIVES

If you're under thirty-five, do not have a family or personal history of breast cancer, and are not considered at risk due to any other significant factor, oral contraceptives will most likely *not* increase your risk of breast cancer. That's because the combination pills used these days are very low dose. Studies from the 1970s and early 1980s may also not apply to women today because they studied the effects of much higher dose pills than what women are on today.

That said, the official warnings in your pill packets will tell you that if you have a family history of breast cancer, a pill containing estrogen can put you at greater risk for developing breast cancer prior to menopause. The warnings will also tell you that if you've been on oral contraceptives longer than eight years and/or began them early, you are considered to be statistically at higher risk for breast cancer. One United States study found that women under age thirty-five who used an estrogen-containing pill for more than ten years increased their risk of breast cancer by about 70 percent compared to women who never took oral contraceptives. There are also studies showing no difference in breast cancer risk between women on the pill for ten years compared with non-pill users, as well as studies showing a decreased risk in pill users after age forty-five (which is potentially very good news). Since less than 2 percent of all breast cancers are diagnosed in women under age thirty-five anyway, the study showing an increased risk really shouldn't rattle you all that much. In the final analysis, you're looking at a very small number. Instead of one in five hundred women developing breast cancer before age thirty-five, that statistic increases it to one in three hundred.

At any rate, if you're concerned about breast cancer and oral contraceptives, you may want to ask your doctor about the progestin-only pill, also called the mini-pill. This pill does not contain any estrogen, which is the culprit ingredient of combination oral contraceptives. For the record, women on oral contraceptives are more at risk for blood clots than breast cancer, and the risk of unwanted pregnancy under age twenty should also be weighed.

Age, as discussed above, of course, is also a factor. Since breast cancer incidence increases with age, using oral contraceptives at an older age can also increase your risk. But, as with hormone replacement therapy, we don't know whether the increase is only age-related or whether oral contraceptives truly contribute to the increase.

What you may find interesting, though, is that all oral contraceptives, whether combination or progestin-only, protect you from ovarian and endometrial cancer. That's because you don't ovulate on oral contraceptives, which gives your ovaries a break. Some experts believe that the lowered risk of ovarian and endometrial cancer compensates for the slight increase in breast cancer in the small groups of women who are at high risk for all three. Of course, if you're one of these women, you'll find little comfort in this argument.

PREGNANCY HISTORY

This is one of the biggest known risk factors in determining your overall risk of breast cancer as far as known risk factors are concerned. A 1751 edition of the *Chambers Encyclopedia* described breast cancer as "a most dread disease, particularly of the celibate and barren." To a large extent, this is still true today.

According to the National Cancer Institute, lesbians are two to three times more likely to develop breast cancer than heterosexual women, while childfree women are 50 percent more likely to develop breast cancer than are women who have given birth before age thirty-five. The earlier you have your first child, the greater the protection. If you bear your first child after age thirty-five, your pregnancy no longer offers you the same protection against breast cancer, unless you decide to breastfeed.

Your pregnancy history can be a paradox in terms of breast cancer risk, since pregnancy induces breast maturation and increases estrogen, thereby promoting breast cancer. For example, the more full-term pregnancies a women has, the lower her risk of developing breast cancer after menopause, but women who've had children may be more likely to get breast cancer before they are thirty-five. It has also been suggested that pregnancy slightly increases your risk of breast cancer in the short term, but reduces your long-term risk. Since most breast cancer is in older women, the result is that pregnancy reduces risk of breast cancer overall.

Breast is best

That's right, breastfeeding for even as short as three months can help protect you from premenopausal breast cancer and possibly help to extend protection after menopause, although the latter is in debate. Although it is a well-documented fact that breastfeeding lowers your risk of breast cancer, it was once believed true only for women who breastfeed at younger ages and for long periods of time. This seemed to explain why Inuit women who lactate continuously from age seventeen to fifty had an even lower rate of breast cancer than Japanese women, another low-risk group. But later studies show that no matter how old you are, breastfeeding helps reduce your risks.

A large study by the University of Wisconsin, published in the *New England Journal of Medicine* in January, 1994, found that women who began nursing in their teens and continued for at least six months reduced their risk of breast cancer by 50 percent, while women in their twenties who nursed for the same period of time reduced their risk by 22 percent.

While researchers are still trying to figure out exactly why breastfeeding protects you from breast cancer, part of the answer may lie in a delay in ovulation (breastfeeding usually delays the return of menstrual cycles for an additional six months after delivery). Breastfeeding hormones, prolactin and oxytocin, may also provide protection and cause potentially beneficial physical changes in the breast. An interesting experiment found that lactating rats and mice were more resistant to the effects of chemical carcinogens when compared with the non-lactating rats and mice. This experiment led researchers to conclude that something about lactation helps the breast eliminate carcinogens by secreting them through the milk. If human lactation bears any resemblance to rodent lactation, then this may be true for us, too. Other research suggests that breastfeeding not only helps clear pesticides from the mother's body, but also lowers the lifetime risk of cancer in the breastfed baby. It is also possible that lactation is necessary to complete breast maturation, thus helping with resistance to things that can cause cancer. Here are more eye-openers: If women who breastfeed for three months were to extend their breastfeeding to four to twelve months, breast cancer rates in premenopausal women with children would drop by a significant 11 percent. That represents a lot of women who would avoid getting breast cancer. And, if all mothers followed the World Health Organization guidelines and breastfed for two years or more, breast cancer incidence in premenopausal women with children would drop by 25 percent. Keep in mind that this rate would drop even further in women who breastfeed for these durations in their teens and twenties. Most interesting was the finding that women who traditionally breastfeed with only one breast are more likely to get breast cancer in the unsuckled breast.

Abortion

If a pregnancy is interrupted through a therapeutic abortion (surgical termination of a pregnancy), some studies indicate that the risks of breast cancer may increase. Here's why.

Once you become pregnant, even if you later terminate the pregnancy, your breasts change in structure. The hormonal symphony that controls pregnancy causes cellular changes in your breasts as well as tissue growth. Your breasts continue to change throughout the pregnancy until reaching their final maturation prior to delivery, when you're physically able to breastfeed. If a pregnancy ends abruptly in the first trimester, all the changes your breasts have been going through suddenly stop, making the cells less stable—and possibly more vulnerable to cancer. Even if subsequent pregnancies go to term, your risk remains slightly increased due to the abortion. Some studies suggest that the more abortions you have, the greater your risk, but this conclusion is highly debatable. Conclusions about abortion and breast cancer risk are divided. There are studies that definitely conclude that induced abortion, regardless of what country it takes place in, or when in the first trimester it takes place, increases your risk of breast cancer. On the other hand, an extremely large study published in the *New England Journal of Medicine* concludes that there is no link between abortion and breast cancer. It's suggested that the discrepancies seem to lie in the fact that women who had breast cancer are more willing to disclose their abortion histories.

In sharp contrast, women who carry their first baby to term reduce their risk of breast cancer by roughly 50 percent. So, all we can say at this point is that women who abort *may* be at greater risk if they're eighteen or under; they're aborting after eight weeks; or breast cancer runs in their family. Interestingly, one study found that women who had abortions but later breastfed a child did not seem to increase their risk of breast cancer.

WEIGHT

As discussed earlier in the diet section, the more fat eaten in your culture, the higher the rate of breast cancer in your cultural group. We don't know if this is

Table 1.2

CALCULATING YOUR RISK

What causes breast cancer? In most cases, experts don't know. Known risk factors may account for less than 70 percent of all cases. This table compares high-risk groups with groups with the lowest risks. Comparing the "relative risks" can be tricky. For example, a 90-percent increase in risk may sound high, but it's less than two times the risk (that would be a 100-percent increase).

If you have:	Your risk is:	Than if you have:

Mother diagnosed with breast
   cancer before age 60
   after age 60
	
	2 times higher
	40% higher
		No first-degree relatives (mother,
		   sister, or daughter) with breast
		   cancer

Two first-degree relatives with breast cancer	 4–6 times higher	
Menarche at age 11–14 at age 15	30% higher 10% higher	Menarche at age 16

First child born at age 20–24
   at age 25–29
   at age 30 or older
   No biological children
	30% higher
	60% higher
	90% higher
	90% higher
		First child born before age 20

Menopause at age 55 or older before age 45	50% higher 30% lower	Menopause at age 45–54

Benign breast disease
   with proliferation
   with atypical hyperplasia
	50% higher
	30% lower
	50% higher
		No biopsy or aspiration for
		   benign disease

Repeated fluoroscopy	50% times higher to 2 times higher	No special exposure
Heaviest 10% of women age 50 or older	20% higher	Thinnest 10% of women'

Tallest 10% of women
   age 30–49
   age 50 or older
	
	30% higher
	40% higher
		Shortest 10% of women

Current use of birth control pills Part use of birth control pills	50% higher No higher	Never used birth control pills

Current use of estrogen
   replacement therapy
   age under 55
   age 55–59
   age 60 or older
Past use of estrogen therapy
	
	20% higher
	50% higher
	2.1 times higher
	No higher
		Never used estrogen replacement
		   therapy

1 alcoholic drink a day 2 drinks a day 3 drinks a day	40% higher 70% higher 2 times higher	No alcoholic beverage use

Source: Nutrition Action Newsletter, *January/February 1996. Adapted from* New England Journal of Medicine *327 (1992): 319.*

due to the fat eaten, or due to other dietary and lifestyle differences among cultures. However, we do know that the more fat on your body, the greater your risk of postmenopausal breast cancer. That may be because fat cells store estrogen and manufacture it, increasing your risk of estrogen-dependent cancers as well as a number of other diseases. By contrast, tall, thin premenopausal women seem to be more at risk for breast cancer than their average height and weight counterparts. Studies also show that women who have gained weight after 35 are more at risk for postmenopausal breast cancer, but this risk drops slightly if you've lost weight after age 18 or 35.

Apples and pears

While we can all do something about our weight, it's difficult to do much about body shape. Unfortunately, one study has actually linked certain body shapes to breast cancer. Apparently, pear-shaped figures are less at risk for breast cancer than apple-shaped figures that carry more weight around the waist than the hips and thighs. Data indicates that the fat in the "spare tire" area is more metabolically active than the fat on the thighs, hips, and rear ends. However, the apple-shape theory was not supported by researchers from the Memorial Sloan-Kettering Cancer Center, who in 1993 reported no such link between body shape and breast cancer. Interestingly, smoking changes fat metabolism so that it is distributed more in the middle (though this may not increase your risk of breast cancer, since smoking is also linked to earlier menopause).

A DISTURBING THEORY: ENVIRONMENTAL ESTROGENS

In 1962, environmentalist Rachel Carson wrote a book called Silent Spring, which essentially said: wake up and smell the chemicals; wildlife and humans are dying from pesticides and pollutants. Carson was denounced by industry and medical leaders as hysterical, and died of breast cancer herself in 1964. Today, many renowned scientists in both the environmental and medical research communities are concluding that maverick Rachel Carson was right all along, including Dr. Theo Colborne, senior scientist at the World Wildlife

Fund, and co-author of Our Stolen Future *(1996), and Dr. Sandra Steingraber, whose book* Living Downstream: An Ecologist Looks at Cancer and the Environment *(1997), is being seen as this generation's* Silent Spring. *Living Downstream is helping the cancer research community to finally accept the disturbing information you're about to read as fact. Dr. Steingraber put it best at a lecture she gave in Toronto: "Science likes to prove the same thing over and over again before it says that something is fact. And that's usually a good thing. But sometimes calling for more research is the grandfather excuse for doing nothing." This sentiment is echoed by the International Joint Commission on the Great Lakes: "Scientific arguments and their lack of absolute proof can also be used as an excuse for inaction. The phrase 'good science' has been used to block change through demands for more rigorous proof." (Eighth Biennial* Report on Great Lakes Water Quality, *1996, p. 17). Indeed, had we waited for clear scientific proof that cigarettes cause lung cancer, we'd still be waiting for that Surgeon General's warning!*

Seventy percent of all women who get breast cancer have none of the known risk factors we hear so much about. But, if hereditary, biological, and behavioral factors are not the largest contributing factors, what are?

Many experts suggest a link between the environment to breast cancer. For example, fallout from above-ground nuclear tests conducted in the 1950s coincide with the current breast cancer statistics in areas contaminated with the fallout. Between 1945 and 1963 over 100 nuclear bomb tests were conducted in the United States alone, not including Russia and China. But the role chemical pollutants play is far more ominous.

Clearly, something has gone terribly wrong in industrialized countries for the incidence of breast cancer (and other cancers) to reach such alarming rates. Some theorize that many of the answers lie in an environmental phenomenon which is beginning to receive increasing attention from traditional medical practitioners.

In 1994, a major discovery led medical researchers and environmental scientists to the same conclusion: Life on planet earth is being affected by a group of substances known as environmental estrogens. A long list of organic chemicals, found in various pesticides and plastics, is transforming in the natural environment into substances that have similar effects to the female hormone estrogen. The results, especially in areas that are highly contaminated, can be very severe for sensitive species. For humans, it's been postulated that environmental estrogens may reduce male sperm count, and possibly contribute to increased rates of reproductive cancers, such as breast cancer in women and testicular cancer in men.

Major players in the discovery of environmental estrogens were Professor Carlos Sonnenschein and Associate Professor Ana Soto, breast cancer researchers at Tufts University School of Medicine in Boston. During routine research using previously obtained cells that had been stored in plastic test tubes, Sonnenschein and Soto were puzzled when they found that the cancer cells had mysteriously grown and divided. Normally, most breast cancer cells are estrogen-receptor positive, meaning that the more estrogen present in the body, the more an estrogen-receptor-positive cancer spreads. This is why anti-estrogen drugs, such as tamoxifen (discussed further in Chapters 4 and 10) have been developed. However, in Sonnenschein's and Soto's experiment, the cancer cells had been deliberately isolated from estrogen. Therefore, the cells should have remained dormant. But instead, the cells behaved as though they were "swimming" in estrogen. After repeating the experiment several times, they found the source of the estrogen effect was the test tube itself. An estrogenic substance was leaching from the plastic test tubes. In a sense, the plastic was "leaking" estrogen into the cells it "housed."

Sonnenschein and Soto explored this bizarre occurrence further. They tracked down the company that manufactured the test tubes, but were denied access to the manufacturer's plastic "recipe." On their own, they tried to isolate the ingredient causing the estrogenic effect. To their horror, they found that the guilty ingredient was *nonylphenol*, which is used in hundreds of everyday consumer products: detergents, toiletries, cosmetics, and oils. It also lines the insides of canned goods; it is found in various plastic food wraps, in spermicides and contraceptive foam, and a variety of other products.

As Sonnenschein and Soto were digging into the plastic side of this estrogen revelation, several experiments were being conducted worldwide that confirmed and reaffirmed their findings. Dr. David Feldman, a researcher at a laboratory in Stanford University, had also stumbled onto the plastic discovery.

Meanwhile, environmental scientists had begun to notice that several wildlife species were developing hermaphroditic traits. In the Florida swamplands, alligators were simply not breeding. A concerned research team from the University of Florida pulled male alligators out of the water to examine their genitals. The majority of male alligators were sterile as a result of either undeveloped or abnormally shaped penises. A chemical spill in nearby waters was found to be the culprit and had an estrogenic effect on the alligators' natural habitat.

Twenty-three hundred kilometers north, in a Canadian creek on Lake Superior, scientists found that fish living in waters close to a pulp mill, which contained certain chemicals with estrogenic effects, were now complete hermaphrodites. The male fish had developed ovaries and were sterile; the female fish had exaggerated ovaries. In other contaminated waters, fish had actually exploded from thyroid hormone overactivity after developing goiters (enlarged thyroid glands).

Swedish and British researchers have been concerned since the late 1980s about the increase in male infertility. More male infants are being born with *cryptorchidism*, a condition in which the testicles do not descend into the scrotum but remain undescended inside the abdomen. One study found a decrease over the last fifty years in the quality of human semen. (Note: A recent study measuring sperm quality in New York City contraindicated these findings.) In Britain, testicular cancer incidence has tripled over the last fifty years; it is now the most common cancer in men under age thirty. For example, in Denmark, there has been a 400 percent increase in testicular cancer. As for prostate cancer, the incidence has doubled over the last decade. It's been suggested that these male reproductive problems have been linked to environmental estrogens, too.

The scientific literature is slowly becoming saturated with studies linking one organic chemical after another to reproductive cancers and endocrine disruption in both wildlife and humans. These studies, from all corners of the world, are reaching the same conclusion: Organic chemicals are transforming into environmental estrogens. Some suggest that environmental estrogens are "feminizing" the planet, and women are perhaps being overloaded with estrogen, which may account for the rise of estrogen-dependent cancers as well as estrogen-related conditions, such as endometriosis and fibroids. Estrogen pollutants are also thought to accumulate in fatty tissues. Since women generally carry more body fat than men, they may be accumulating more of these toxins. Many studies have found that women with breast cancer have greater concentrations of DDT in their breast fat or blood samples than women without breast cancer. In fact, exposure to DDT has been linked to a risk of breast cancer that is two to ten times greater than women who have not been exposed.

Research at Cornell University suggests that there is a "good" and "bad" estrogen similar to good and bad cholesterol; bad estrogen can trigger breast cancer cell growth. It's thought that estrogenic pesticides "stack the deck" with bad estrogen somehow. Studies have shown that human breast cancer cells had four times the amount of "bad estrogen" than normal breast cells. In the future, blood tests may be able to measure "good" and "bad" estrogen

The picture may be equally dismal for men, who may be slowly sterilized by this phenomenon and are also developing reproductive cancers. Several prominent scientists have gone on record to say that this problem is *the* environmental priority of the next century.

On the flip side, many doctors point out a huge increase in the obesity of the Western world's population. This also increases the level of estrogen produced by our bodies. Plants are also a source of natural hormones—phytoestrogens (as well as anti-estrogens).

DDT: BANNED BUT NOT FORGOTTEN

Pesticides are major contributors to this environmental estrogen problem, one of the most notorious of which is DDT. DDT stands for dichloro-diphenyl-trichlore-ethane and was formally banned in most industrialized countries by the mid-1970s. It was discovered in the late nineteenth century by a German chemist, but wasn't considered an insecticide until 1939, when Switzerland's

Paul Mueller won a Nobel Prize for its new-found use. DDT was considered a godsend to the agricultural world.

DDT was banned in North America because it was essentially wreaking havoc on several wildlife species. DDT is considered to be an estrogen pollutant when it breaks down into its byproduct DDE. Until recently, no one really understood why DDT seemed to target reproductive systems, but with the discovery of environmental estrogens, the mystery is apparently solved. Unfortunately, even though DDT is banned in North America, it is still in use in other parts of the world. While some experts wonder whether DDT is the reason why breast and other cancers are rising in the developing world, it is only one of many possible factors, such as changes in pregnancy age, number of children, and breastfeeding habits.

Even though DDT has been pretty much banned in most countries since 1972, it remains active in the environment for twenty-five to thirty years.

There is some promising news, however. Health Canada found that DDT levels in breastmilk dropped from roughly 150 parts per billion (ppb) in 1967 to less than 15 ppb in 1986, and they are still falling. PCBs, which are also banned in North America, fell from 30 ppb to about 5 ppb in Canada, while the Environmental Protection Agency reports that PCB levels in Lake Michigan trout dropped from 23 parts per million in 1974 to 3 parts per million in 1993—still 2 parts per million above the safety limit, though.

IT'S A TOXIC, TOXIC WORLD

A variety of exotic chemical concoctions exist abundantly in the air. Organochlorines are particularly nasty; they are persistent in the environment and are fat soluble in the bodies of wildlife and humans. Organochlorines such as DDT, DDE, dioxins, and PCBs (polychlorinated biphenyls) have accumulated and concentrated in the food chain.

A 1987 study identified 177 organochlorines in the fat, breast milk, blood, semen, and breath of the general North American population. It's estimated that billions of gallons of these toxic substances have been released into an environment ill-equipped to cope with them. Since these chemicals are resistant to breaking down, they're spread through the air and water, exposing humans to these poisons in our food, groundwater, surface water, and air. According to a 1992 Greenpeace report on chlorine and human health, no industrial organochlorines are known to be non-toxic.

A brief history of manmade chemicals

Although PCBs were first introduced into the environment in 1929, large scale production of manmade chemicals started only after World War II. By 1947, the United States was producing 259,000 pounds of pesticides annually; by 1960, 636.7 million pounds of pesticides were being produced. In terms of synthetic fibers, between 1945 and 1970, the production increased by almost 6,000 percent; plastics production increased by almost 2,000 percent; nitrogen fertilizers and synthetic organic chemicals increased by about 1,000 percent; organic solvents increased by 746 percent. Industry now produces roughly forty million tons of chlorine per year to make products such as plastic, solvents, pesticides, and refrigerants. After that, thousands of organochlorines occur as byproducts, particularly in the pulp and paper industry. These chemicals are spread by wind and water, sprayed on plants, or ingested by animals we eat and settle in our fat and tissues.

WHAT SHOULD YOU DO?

Although some of this information has been peppering the headlines over the last couple of years, much of it is news to many of you. There are a number of lifestyle changes you can make to limit your exposure to these toxins. There are also a number of things you can do to pressure industry and government into waking up and smelling the estrogenic toxins. This topic is discussed in detail in Chapter 10.

HOT ZONES

A number of studies have identified industry and community pockets where breast cancer incidence is higher. How much does this have to do with industry? Women working in the petroleum and chemical industries have significantly higher rates of breast cancer than the general public. Rates of breast cancer are roughly 6.5 times higher in United States counties with chemical waste sites than in counties where no waste sites exist. A study published in 1991 on 1,583 dioxin-exposed German workers revealed that the rate of breast cancer doubled. Again, there may have been other factors that weren't considered, such as age, lifestyle, pregnancy history, and socio-economic status.

Another study in 1991, published in the *American Journal of Industrial Medicine,* examined occupational exposure to a variety of toxins and cancer incidence in the state of New Jersey. The study looked at 17,621 cancer cases that had been collected by the New Jersey State Cancer Registry between 1979 and 1984. The results showed that breast cancer incidence was higher in women working in both the chemical and pharmaceutical industries, while breast cancer mortality rates were higher in the electrical and printing industries. The study also found higher rates of uterine cancer for women in several manufacturing industries, including rubber and plastic products, apparel, and electrical equipment.

One of the most well-known breast cancer hot zones is Long Island, New York, where the organization 1 in 9 and the Long Island Breast Cancer Action Coalition are based. By the 1980s, Long Island's breast cancer rate was 110.6 per 100,000 women compared with the national rate of 94.7 per 100,000. This higher rate was thought to be associated with environmental toxins found in Long Island waste-disposal sites, commuter car exhaust, electromagnetic fields, polluted drinking water, and over eight hundred chemical plants in that area. This higher breast cancer rate led to a study conducted by the New York State Health Department, which was released in mid-1994. Disturbingly, it showed that women living near large chemical plants had a significantly greater risk of developing breast cancer after menopause than women who didn't. However, many scientists argued that this study did not prove a definite association between breast cancer and chemical plants, only a possible association.

The bottom line is that where there is heavy industry, there are higher cancer rates of all kinds. In the United States, the Northeastern states comprise the five highest cancer mortality rates in the United States; while the rural Western and Southern states comprise the five lowest cancer mortality rates.

In Canada, Ontario has higher cancer rates than other parts of Canada. In Europe, England has the highest cancer mortality rates in the world, while southern Italy has exceptionally low cancer mortality rates.

WHEN SHOULD YOU GO FOR RISK COUNSELING?

Breast cancer is one of the diseases women most fear. And it seems as though another study finds yet another possible factor that *may* be linked to breast cancer. Therefore, risk counseling has emerged as an option for women who can't seem to make sense of the conflicting information regarding risk. (It may not be available everywhere, however, since it's an emerging field.)

Breast cancer risk analysis entails having your family history, lifestyle, and genetic predispositions analyzed by a breast cancer risk expert. Most of these experts have a background in genetic counseling, but they are not necessarily medical doctors. By the end of one session, which costs roughly U.S. $350 as of 1996 (not insured), you'll be told that your chances of developing breast cancer at a given age are X or Y percent. For example, you might be told that if you live to age seventy-five, your lifetime risk is about 7 percent.

A 1994 *Vogue* article pointed out that sometimes the analysis can conflict with a doctor's advice. In one instance, a counselor had seen two women with fibrocycstic breast condition (discussed in Chapter 2) and a family history of breast cancer. Both women had been advised by their physicians to have preventive mastectomy performed. However, since only a rare form of fibrocycstic breast condition, which neither woman had, leads to breast cancer—and even then only about 10 percent of the time—the risk counselor felt a mastectomy was unnecessary at that point.

This kind of analysis may prove helpful for women seeking a second, very independent opinion. Ideally, your doctor or any breast surgeon can also do a risk analysis. The problem is that many simply don't have time, though this may change in the very near future.

ARE YOU A CUSTOMER?

Since most women grossly overestimate their risk of breast cancer by as much as four times, it's probably worth the money to have some peace of mind and a more realistic perspective if you're worried about it. Again, if you're looking for answers solely based on known risk factors, you probably won't get much more than you would from a tea leaf reading. Again, 70 percent of the women who develop breast cancer do not have any of the known risk factors. In the meantime, use the following guidelines to help you make your decision about counseling:

You have reason to worry about breast cancer before age fifty if:
1. You have a first-degree relative (mother or sister) who had/has breast cancer prior to age fifty particularly if she had cancer in both breasts prior to menopause.
2. You yourself had breast, ovarian, uterine, endometrial, or colon cancer (all estrogen-dependent).
3. You've been exposed to high levels of radiation to your chest area (exposure from fluoroscopy, other high-dose medical X rays, or nuclear fallout). Mammography and normal low-dose diagnostic chest X rays *don't count.*
4. You're a DES daughter (minor risk).
5. You did not breastfeed.

You have reason to worry about breast cancer after age fifty if:
1. You have a first-degree relative (mother, sister, or daughter) who has or had breast cancer.
2. You have a first-degree relative (mother, sister, or daughter) who has or had colon, ovarian, or endometrial cancer.
3. You yourself had breast cancer, colon, ovarian, or endometrial cancer.
4. You've been exposed to high levels of radiation to your chest area (exposure from fluoroscopy, other high-dose medical X rays, or nuclear fallout). Mammography and normal low-dose diagnostic chest X rays don't count.

5. You have dense breast tissue (more problems with interpreting mammogram results).
6. You have had breast biopsies done for benign breast problems, excluding fibroadenomas (discussed further in Chapter 2).
7. You had early menarche (first period at an early age).
8. You did not breastfeed (minor risk).
9. You are obese or eat large amounts of fat (minor risk).
10. You have never been pregnant (minor risk).
11. You are a DES daughter (minor risk).

You MAY have reason to worry about breast cancer before or after age fifty if:
1. You have high estrogen levels (shown on a blood test).
2. You have more years of education than average (there are some cultural/lifestyle risks associated with this).
3. You don't eat many fruits, vegetables, soy, or sea vegetables.
4. You live in a highly industrialized area with chemical plants nearby.
5. You're exposed to estrogenic chemicals in your workplace or home (see pages 15–16 above).
6. You're overweight.

No matter how old you are, if your fear of breast cancer is interfering with your quality of life, consider risk counseling, or make an appointment with your doctor to discuss your risk profile.

· · · · · · ·

As discussed in the Introduction, good nutrition and disease prevention is covered in the last chapter. That's because most of us will want to get down to the "nuts and bolts" of breast health and breast cancer *first*. The next chapter deals with how the breast works, good breast health, breast screening, investigating suspicious lumps, and a hundred other things that might make you ask: Is it cancer?

CHAPTER 2

IS IT CANCER?

If you're like me, a common "daymare" (by this, I mean a daydreamed night-mare) is being in the bath or shower and finding a lump in my breast. I some-times think the fear of that moment has a worse effect than the lump itself. But the way to lessen the fear is not to ignore your breasts or to pray that day never comes, it is to find out everything you can about normal breast anatomy, func-tion, and breast conditions that are common but harmless. This chapter dis-cusses: how breasts were designed to work, a variety of harmless breast conditions, infections in non-lactating and lactating women, investigating lumps, and routine screening methods, as well as ways to maximize various screening methods such as BSE and mammography.

HOW YOUR BREAST WORKS

Most of us grew up with little information about how our breasts mature and work. But in order to understand how breast cancer develops, it is essential to have this knowledge.

Technically breasts exist to produce milk to feed babies, but anthropolo-gists believe that breasts serve another important purpose: they attract and arouse males—crucial for reproduction. It is breasts that define our biological class; the word *mammal* comes from *mammary gland*—which is what the breast is. Although breasts of mammals vary in size and number, human females are the only biological group that develops full breasts long before they're needed for breastfeeding. This phenomenon has to do with the fact that we can engage in sex when we are not fertile. When a woman's nipple is stimulated during lovemaking, the hormone oxytocin is released. Oxytocin is responsible for milk "let down" in lactating women, for labor contractions in pregnant women, and for uterine contractions that enhance orgasm in women who are neither pregnant nor breastfeeding.

Human breast tissue begins to develop in the sixth week of fetal life. The "milk ridge," a line from the armpit all the way down to the groin, develops at this point. In most cases, by the ninth week, the milk ridge is only in the chest area, but both women and men can develop accessory nipples (these look like moles to the untrained eye) and even breast tissue all the way down to the groin. (Other mammals retain the milk ridge, which is why they have multiple nipples.) And since the mother's sex hormones have been circulating through the placenta, both girls and boys are sometimes born with little breasts.

In girls, nothing much happens to the breasts until puberty, when the pituitary gland starts the entire reproductive and development cycle. Puberty is triggered when the follicle stimulating hormone (FSH) stimulates the ovary to produce estrogen and progesterone at ovulation. Pubic hair develops at this time, generally before breasts appear, but it could happen the other way around.

Breasts begin to develop at this point, too. Their development comprises five stages. In the prepubertal stage, the nipple becomes slightly more prominent. In the breast bud stage, breasts begin to develop. During the third stage, breast elevation, the breast is formed and becomes more erect; in the fourth stage, the areolar mound, the areola enlarges in circumference. The last stage, the adult contour, occurs when the breast is mature enough to produce milk. The menstrual period is usually the finale to the breast's initial development. Further breast development occurs during pregnancy, which has become the focus of intensive research to find out why pregnancy (especially early pregnancy) tends to reduce the risk of breast cancer.

Breasts are considered to have reached maturity when they are capable of breastfeeding, but the breast isn't considered fully *functional* until lactation begins.

BREAST ENGINEERING

In medicalspeak, the breast is a secretory gland because it secretes fluid—milk. In order to produce milk, the breast relies on other organs: glandular tissue, which both produces and transports milk; connective tissue, which supports the breast so that it sits in an upright position; arterial blood supply, which not only nourishes the breast tissue, but delivers the nutrients essential for the breast to make milk; and the venous and lymphatic systems, which remove waste. (Lymph nodes are part of the lymphatic system, which are like little POW camps that hold and "interrogate" foreign invaders, a topic I discuss in greater detail in the following pages.)

Figure 2.1

WHAT'S INSIDE YOUR BREAST

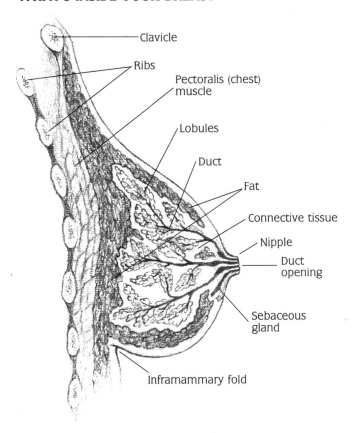

The breast is also made from a hefty amount of fatty tissue (called adipose tissue), which protects the breast from injury. The amount of fatty tissue determines the size of the breast, but has absolutely no effect on a woman's ability to lactate. See figure 2.1.

How lactation works

During lactation, the breast relies on alveoli (pronounced al-vee-oh-lie), grape-like clusters of glandular tissue that help to make milk out of blood. Alveoli cells are surrounded by a layer of bandlike cells called myoepithelial cells. If you imagine a real cluster of grapes, the myoepithelial cells are the grape skin, while the alveoli cells are the juicy grapes lying just beneath the skin. When stimulated by oxytocin, the myoepithelial cells contract around the alveoli cells, expelling the milk into the ductules and the milk ducts. Imagine a real grape between your fingers. When you squeeze the grape, it will squirt juice all over your hand. Oxytocin is the "squeeze" that makes the alveoli's milk squirt out.

And how does the milk come out of the nipple? Well, like an automatic coffee maker, your breasts are fully equipped with a "transport" system that delivers the breast's liquids right down a baby's throat. Extending from the alveoli are branch-like tubes called ductules. Each of these ductules empties into larger ducts called mammary ducts (a.k.a. lactiferous ducts). Picture those grape clusters again. Now, imagine them still on the vine. The tiny branches leading to the stem would be the ductules, while the main stem connecting each grape cluster is the mammary duct. Each of these "stems" leads to the nipple.

Just before they reach the nipple, the mammary ducts swell and widen underneath the nipple and areola (the darker area of pigment surrounding the nipple) to become lactiferous sinuses. This is where the milk collects and waits for a baby to start suckling. The sinus narrows to an opening in the nipple (called a nipple pore).

Going back to the grape vine analogy, several clusters of grapes are connected to a single stem. Well, within the breast, each of these stems forms a lobe. There are fifteen to twenty-five lobes in the breast, and each lobe consists of twenty to forty lobules (a smaller milk duct with its supporting alveoli). Each lobule consists of ten to a hundred supporting alveoli. It's a little like that wooden Ukrainian doll game: Open up a lobe, and you find a smaller lobe identical to it; open up the smaller lobe, and you find an even smaller one.

The parts you can actually see

Finally, we come to the nipple. All mammary ducts lead directly to the nipple. Some mammary ducts merge near the very tip of the nipple. Thanks to the delicate nerve endings, the nipple tissue is extremely sensitive. When it is touched or stimulated, it protrudes and becomes firmer. The nipple is also designed to be flexible and easily manipulated so it can fit into a baby's mouth during breastfeeding.

The darker area that surrounds the nipple, called the areola (pronounced airy-olah), also houses the Montgomery glands, which act as tiny muscles that contract and widen to help get the milk out during lactation. The Montgomery glands also produce oils that lubricate the nipple and discourage the growth of bacteria on the skin of the nipple and the areola during lactation. It is the Montgomery glands that enlarge during pregnancy, giving the areola a knobbly appearance. For information on the pregnant and postpartum breast, consult my books *The Pregnancy Sourcebook* and *The Breastfeeding Sourcebook.*

HARMLESS BREAST CONDITIONS

Breasts are complex glands made up of fat, connective tissue, lobes, ductules, ducts, and so on. Because they're ultrasensitive to the pituitary hormones that command the reproductive cycle, there are numerous breast conditions women develop that have nothing to do with cancer and everything to do with normal life with breasts. Unfortunately, many clinical labels brand a woman as having a breast disease when, in fact, all she has is a perfectly natural breast responding to natural occurrences—be it hormones, bruises, or bacteria. Lumpy breasts and infections, which I discuss in the following section, are nothing to panic about.

FIBROCYSTIC BREAST DISEASE: AN OUTDATED DIAGNOSIS

Many women are diagnosed with a breast condition called fibrocystic breast disease. The term evolved in the premammography era and was used by pathologists (doctors who study tissue) to describe a wide variety of breast conditions they came across when examining breast tissue biopsies. Biopsies at this time were done for breast lumps, breast pain, and "thickening" or "nodularity." When higher resolution mammograms became widely available as a diagnostic tool, the term *fibrocystic disease* stuck and moved into mainstream practice. As a result, any time women had breast pain, breast lumps, or breast cysts, they were diagnosed with fibrocystic disease—which not only sounds far more ominous than it is, but also stigmatized health insurance policies. As soon as insurers saw *fibrocystic breast disease* on a policy-holder's charts, they rated premiums higher or wanted to drop the policy.

To solve the problem, a committee of the College of American Pathologists met in 1985 to discuss changing the diagnostic term "fibrocystic breast disease" to "fibrocystic breast *condition*." Many other non-specific medical terms were revised for specification at this time, too.

What if you're still diagnosed with fibrocystic breast disease?

This is a sign that your doctor is *way* behind the times. Either ask your doctor to define what s/he means by disease (is it lumpy/bumpy breasts or cyclical breast pain) and request that "disease" be upgraded to "condition" on your charts, or get yourself to a doctor that is familiar with the current terminology. For the record, when you have "lumpy/bumpy" breasts, you have fibrocystic condition (discussed next). These lumps may become more exaggerated around your period, which is simply a normal response to hormonal changes.

FIBROCYSTIC CONDITION

Okay. You've been diagnosed with fibrocystic condition. What does this mean? First, it does not mean that you're going to develop breast cancer. Doctors use it to describe a number of separate and distinct breast conditions that have nothing to do with each other. These conditions range from normal breast tenderness that develops before your period to fibroadenomas and cysts.

If you have any of the following breast conditions, please remember that none of them cause breast cancer, although, on rare occasions, some of them are signs of certain breast cancers.

1. *Tender breasts associated with PMS.* If you suffer from premenstrual "tender boobs," join the club. Tenderness is a normal physiological condition that occurs during or before your period, along with swelling and

lumpiness (due to water retention). Unfortunately, a disturbing trend in medicine is to diagnose premenstrual breast pain as a "sickness." So instead of comforting and reassuring women about what is physiologically normal, some doctors seem to be manufacturing illnesses around normal occurrences in the female body.

So "cyclical breast pain," as PMS-breast tenderness is often called, is never a sign of breast cancer. Some women report that eliminating caffeine from their diet can alleviate PMS breast tenderness, but no study has proven that this is absolutely helpful. What *does* help to relieve breast tenderness is evening primrose oil, which you'll find at most drug stores or health food stores. Breast specialists recommend that, once your breast pain is evaluated to rule out a more serious condition, you try evening primrose oil for three months to see if it works; many women have also had success with vitamin E. The problem with finding a definite therapy for this type of breast pain is that it generally goes away on its own in response to the hormonal cycle; as a result, it does decrease, if not disappear, after menopause. For more information on PMS symptoms, consult my book, *The Gynecological Sourcebook.*

2. *Non-cyclical breast pain.* Also known as chronic mastalgia (or breast pain), non-cyclical breast pain is anatomical, that is, it is not hormones but something inside the breast itself that causes the pain, which is why the pain does not necessarily disappear with menopause like hormonal or PMS-linked breast pain. Often, this pain is caused by a large cyst—in fact, many women are prone to painful cysts.

Non-cyclical breast pain can also result from a bruise and is very, very rarely an indication of cancer. Your gynecologist or primary care physician should check to find the source of the pain and should also be able to relieve the pain (by aspirating a cyst, for example). If the doctor is unable to locate the source of the pain or prescribe relief for it, see an experienced breast specialist who will take a careful history, perform a careful physical exam (versus a breast "pat" that takes two seconds), and may recommend a mammogram.

3. *Non-breast-origin pain.* This type of pain that has nothing to do with your breasts. Non-breast-origin pain can result from a form of arthritis called costochondritis, which can be diagnosed by a breast specialist.. Men get this pain too, and sometimes mistake it for a heart attack, while women who experience such pain tend to suspect breast cancer. You will need to be treated for arthritic pain to relieve it. A pinched nerve in the neck or a type of phlebitis (inflamed vein) in the breast can also cause breast pain. These conditions cure themselves over time.

4. *Infections and inflammations.* Breast infections are discussed on page 52.

5. *Discharge and other nipple problems.* Discharge should not be confused with secretions, which are pretty common. The difference is that discharge comes out of the nipple on its own, without any suction or pressure. As for secretions, one study found that 83 percent of women of all ages and lactation histories had secretions when their breasts were gently suctioned— even if they weren't lactating. Basically, discharge occurs when prolactin gets activated and tells the brain to send down fluid in a confused instinct. Although some BSE (breast self-exam) pamphlets will tell you to squeeze the nipple for discharge, and some doctors will routinely squeeze the nipple during examinations, the fluid that comes out is a secretion that is usually normal and is caused by the squeezing itself. The only time you should worry is when nipple discharge occurs by itself and comes out of one breast only. This condition is usually caused by an infection, but it can also be a sign of cancer in about 4 percent of cases and warrants a visit to the doctor. Fluid from your nipple can be analyzed for signs of atypical cells.

   Nipples can also get itchy due to rashes, dry skin, or eczema. The condition is discussed in detail on page 57. In rare cases, a kind of breast skin cancer known as Paget's disease can occur. Paget's disease responds well to treatment.

In summary, whether you're diagnosed with fibrocystic condition or fibrocystic breast disease, you should ask your doctor what specific breast symptoms led him or her to this conclusion and what therapy he or she recommends. Then, refer to the list above and calm down.

INFECTIONS

Breasts and nipples are like any other part of the body: they can also get infected. Antibiotics will fix the infection. Infections generally occur in breastfeeding women.

LACTATIONAL MASTITIS

This is an infection of the milk-producing breast which happens during breast-feeding. The condition affects as many 10 percent of breastfeeding women and occurs when bacteria (usually staphylococcus, sometimes streptococcus, both normal skin bacteria we all carry around) gets inside the breast through the nipple. Lactational mastitis sometimes occurs after a milk duct becomes plugged. Plugged ducts (discussed later) may or may not be associated with mastitis, however. In other words, plugged ducts can occur when you don't have mastitis, but are sometimes a symptom of mastitis.

Before the days of antibiotics and short post-delivery hospital stays, mastitis often became an epidemic that would usually be dealt with in the hospital. Today, mastitis no longer spreads in epidemic proportions due to a radical change in postpartum health practices.

The initial symptoms of mastitis are fatigue and a flu-like muscular aching. This is usually followed by a fever, a rapid pulse, and the development of a hot, reddened, and tender area on the breast. Sore nipples are not a symptom of mastitis, although it is possible to have sore nipples and mastitis. Fever and chills are generally signs that the mastitis is severe and that it is taking your entire body to fight off the infection.

If mastitis isn't treated properly, you may develop an abscess. When a "walled-off" portion of the breast gets bluish red, swollen, and inflamed, this is a classic sign that an abscess is in the making. The abscess would need to be drained with a needle or a tiny incision in the breast. What happens is that your immune system "walls off" the infectious area, allowing the rest of your body to carry on as usual.

Mastitis usually occurs in only one breast, but it is not unusual to see a double-breast infection. In some cases, mastitis affects the composition of the milk, increasing levels of sodium and chloride—probably the body's way of protecting the baby from infection.

Mastitis generally occurs five weeks into breastfeeding and lasts between two to four days if it is treated. It's crucial not to stop breastfeeding when you have mastitis because this can lead to an abscess (discussed further on).

There are three kinds of lactational mastitis. Cellulitis is an inflammation of the cellular breast tissue which occurs when bacteria enters the breast through a break in the skin (usually through a cracked nipple). It is usually seen in the first weeks of breastfeeding.

Adenitis means inflammation of the ducts within the breast. Here, the infection starts in the milk ducts due to poor emptying of a part of the breast, resulting in milk "stasis," where the milk stays inside longer than it should, making pus formation more likely.

Subclinical mastitis is mild mastitis. There are usually no symptoms other than a low fever; you may feel like you have a touch of flu.

NON-LACTATIONAL MASTITIS

This is a bacterial breast infection in non-lactating women. Bacteria somehow gets deeper inside the breast via the ducts in the nipples. Diabetic women are particularly prone to this condition for the same reason that they are for yeast infections (see the section on nipple infections). Usual symptoms are skin boils on the breast and a flu-like feeling. The same antibiotics used to treat lactational mastitis are used here (see the treatment section that follows).

Abscesses

If you have lactational mastitis, the best way to prevent an abscess is to continue to breastfeed frequently, sore side first. The rules for preventing abscess (and managing mastitis) are: heat, rest, empty breast—heat from warm compresses or a warm shower; rest means going to bed and staying there until you feel better (you take baby with you, by the way); emptying the breast means breastfeeding frequently. After nursing, you should express milk from the sore area (a.k.a. "stripping") to see if there's any pus in it; if there is, express milk after each nursing until the milk runs clear. If you do this, an abscess should not develop, and you may not even require antibiotics. It's also important to change positions frequently during feeding. This will help to empty all the milk sinuses and ductules in the breast.

If an abscess does occur, after it is walled off, it will look like a localized, white area just under the surface of the skin which feels very warm and tender when you touch it. Treatment with antibiotics and possibly drainage of the abscess (by means of an incision) may be necessary.

On rare occasions, an abscess may cause a pus-like discharge from your nipple. In any event, once the infection clears (and it will), you should be able to carry on as usual.

Treating mastitis

Depending on how severe your symptoms are, antibiotics may be necessary. For cellulitis, any antibiotic that can handle staphylococcus and is safe to use during breastfeeding is fine. For adenitis, the drug of choice is erythromycin because it penetrates into the milk spaces which are infected (penicillin and ampicillin used to be the old standbys, but many strains of staphylococcus are now resistant to them). In lactational mastitis, antibiotics and continued breastfeeding will cure the infection within 48 hours.

If your mastitis symptoms seem to be less severe, antibiotics may not be necessary.

PLUGGED DUCTS

If you're lactating and develop a sore lump in one area of the breast but don't seem to have a fever, you probably have a plugged duct, also known as a "plug." This usually refers to ducts plugged at the nipple level by thickened milk, but a plug can also occur higher up in the breast, usually due to scarring or breast construction. A higher plug is referred to as an obstructed duct.

In both cases, the soreness occurs because a duct isn't draining properly and has therefore become inflamed. Pressure builds up behind the plug,

Figure 2.2
BLOCKED DUCT

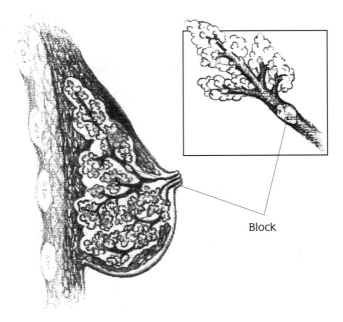

Block

causing inflammation in the surrounding tissues as well. This is also sometimes referred to as "caking," and it usually occurs in only one breast. A milk duct will plug up when milk sits around in the ducts too long as a result of engorgement, breast constriction, or insufficient breast-emptying. The result may be that less milk flows out of the nipple.

In essence, many of the triggers of mastitis (discussed earlier) are at work here, but some women just seem to be prone to chronic plugs; for reasons we don't know, plugged ducts often *cause* mastitis. What we do know is that women tend to be plagued by plugs during winter, probably due to heavier and more restrictive clothing.

Plugged ducts are treated the same way as lactational mastitis: heat, rest, empty breast. In addition, massaging the breast, especially during a hot shower or bath, will help to stimulate the flow of milk.

NIPPLE INFECTIONS

Yeast or bacteria can get into the nipple and cause impetigo (a bacterial infection) or thrush (a yeast infection). Both infections can cause symptoms of burning and irritation. Your doctor can usually tell by your symptoms which kind of infection you have and will prescribe the appropriate medication. If the infection doesn't clear up, your doctor will culture the infection.

Yeast

When yeast occurs in the mouth or nipple, it is called thrush. The two organisms usually responsible for yeast infection are Candida albicans (which causes vaginal yeast infections as well) and Monilia. Both organisms like warm, sweet places and can be transferred from the mouth of a baby or lover to your nipples. When sore nipples erupt suddenly, thrush is the likely cause.

One of the classic triggers of yeast infections is antibiotics. In fact, if you've been treated for mastitis with antibiotics, you may wind up with thrush a few days later. Diabetics (yeast love sugar) and women with a compromised immune system (due to illness or HIV) are also very vulnerable to thrush.

To treat thrush, 1 percent miconozole cream is usually prescribed. The cream must be worked well into the nipple (before and after nursing if you're breastfeeding) to relieve the burning. If a breastfeeding baby also has thrush, this cream will get into the baby's mouth during nursing and will cure the baby, too.

If you seem to be continuously plagued by yeast, you may need to adjust your diet; anemia is a common cause of chronic yeast because it impairs your immune system. Consult your doctor about this. Diet adjustment is a common preventive measure against chronic vaginal yeast, too. You can refer to my book, *The Gynecological Sourcebook*, for more information on chronic yeast infections.

Chronic subareolar abscess

This is an uncommon infection of the sebaceous glands around the nipples. Bacteria is the culprit again; it gets inside the glands during breastfeeding or suckling during lovemaking. The glands get blocked and your breasts get red and form painful boils. This is an unsettling sight, but quite treatable. The glands need to be surgically opened to prevent the infection from recurring. A course of antibiotics and minor breast surgery are the preferred treatments.

Rashes

Nipples are covered with skin, which, like skin anywhere else on your body, can get dry, cracked, and itchy. This can happen due to rashes, dry skin, or even eczema (if you have eczema on other parts of your body, for example). The most common rash is caused by breastfeeding— the frequent skin contact between the baby's mouth and your nipple, perhaps even the solid foods your baby is eating, irritates your nipples. This is a rash that rarely needs medical treatment and clears up if the nipple is kept clean and dry and exposed to sunlight. If a mild rash or dry skin persists, a doctor should be consulted. There is a rare kind of breast cancer called Paget's disease that is characterized by a rash or dryness usually around one nipple.

If the rash on the nipple causes scaling on other areas of the breast, and you notice scaling on other body parts such as the scalp, elbows, or knees, you definitely need to see a doctor to rule out psoriasis. Psoriasis is usually treated with a topical cream containing 1 percent hydrocortisone which is used between feedings and wiped off before breastfeeding.

If you have nipple damage of some kind, Raynaud's syndrome can develop, in which the nipple turns white and is extremely painful during and after feedings. The cure consists of locating the source of the damage (usually a bad latch) and fixing it. A painkiller that is safe to use during breastfeeding will help until the nipples heal.

Breast herpes

If you've been exposed to the herpes simplex virus (HSV), you can develop herpes sores on your nipples. Most doctors will be able to tell if you have a herpes simplex sore (called a vesicle) just by looking at it, but a culture should be done to confirm it.

HSV I and II are now associated with sores above the waist. (In the past,

HSV II was believed to occur only in the genital area). Cold sores and fever blisters are signs that HSV is active. The nipple and areola can also become sites for the sores. (If you're breastfeeding, you may need to wean your baby until the virus has cleared up).

Herpes sores must be kept dry. Dusting them with cornstarch and blow drying them may be helpful for lactating women. There is no cure for herpes, but the sores generally go away and reappear less and less until you will simply not be bothered by them anymore.

The bleb

In rare cases, lactating women may notice a whitish, tender area (bleb) under their areola which looks like milk under the skin. In fact, it is caused by milk somehow becoming trapped there and causing the nipple and areola to become inflamed. The condition causes a lot of pain during breastfeeding and can take several days or weeks to heal. Time is the cure for blebs; you need to wait for the old skin to be replaced by new skin—the bleb is exposed as the old skin cells slough off.

In the meantime, your doctor may need to aspirate the bleb with a fine needle. Or, you can ask for a painkiller. Ice packs in combination with painkillers are the usual route. A topical antibiotic may also be necessary, and often speeds up healing.

LUMPS AND BUMPS

All women are vulnerable to a variety of lumps and bumps in their breasts, the majority of which are benign (harmless or non-cancerous). Unfortunately, though, even a harmless lump is called a tumor in medicalspeak—the word comes from the Latin *tumere*, which means to swell. Tumor simply refers to a clump of primitive cells that are growing and reproducing and forming a lump of some sort. Whether or not the lump is visible depends on where the cells are growing. The primitive cells are divided into two categories: benign and malignant (cancerous). Benign cells are harmless; they don't serve any purpose. If you did nothing at all to remove these cells, they would do nothing more than take up space. They are peaceful in nature and pose no threat to your health.

Malignant cells are "willful," and if left unsupervised, they metastasize (invade) into your organs, taking over them, and causing a lot of damage. They are militant, or "warlike," in nature and mean cancer.

If there was any way doctors could automatically tell a malignant lump from a benign lump, it would relieve much of the anxiety over lumps. Unfortunately, there isn't any way of knowing instantly what the lumps "intentions" are. So *all* suspicious lumps need to be investigated. This is done through various diagnostic procedures that can include needle biopsies, tissue biopsies via stereotactic core needles, lumpectomies (surgically removing the lump), and various imaging procedures such as mammography, where the lump can be photographed and studied more closely.

It is the outcome of these tumor investigations that will tell you whether or not you have cancer. One purpose of this section is tell you all about the investigation process itself and discuss benign tumors in detail.

FATTY TISSUE: THY NAME IS WOMAN

Women have a higher concentration of fat on their bodies, and all kinds of lumps and bumps will form in fatty areas. But these lumps are not usually cancerous. Potentially cancerous lumps are usually found on the breasts, under the arms, or around the neck, which is why it's important to get them investigated as soon as possible.

Lumps around the neck area can be signs of leukemia or Hodgkin's disease, or can indicate malignancies in the throat, thyroid gland, or even lungs. If breast cancer has advanced, it is possible for lumps in the neck (around the collar bone) to form as well.

Breast lumps are frightening, but most of the time they're not cancerous. Most breasts are "lumpy" because of what they're made of: fatty tissue and glandular tissue (glandular tissue is like a bunch of grapes). The problem is, most women don't know the difference between a "normal" lump and a suspicious lump. A normal lump is one that's there for a good reason. A suspicious lump is one that needs to be investigated further because it has characteristics of potentially malignant cells. But in fact, most suspicious breast lumps are not cancerous.

Enlarged lymph nodes that disappear (never suspicious)

Breasts are made up of fat, milk glands, and fibrous supporting tissue. Lymph nodes are also scattered throughout and extend to under the arms. Lymph nodes are like small POW camps set up in the fatty, fleshy areas of our bodies. They work in partnership with the immune system and are designed to capture any kind of suspicious cell that roams near their "camp." A virus will make these "camps" active; when you're healthy, the camps close down. When foreign cells are captured, they're held in the camp for questioning and are then destroyed. So an enlarged or swollen lymph node simply indicates that the nodes have prisoners and are filled up. (Any time you have a cold, for example, the lymph nodes will swell up.)

When you can't feel your lymph nodes at all, it's because there aren't any foreign cells around to keep them open at the moment. Does this mean you need to be actually sick with a virus or cold for a lymph node to swell? No, not at all. We're constantly being invaded with viruses that we're not even aware of. Lymph nodes can fill up with prisoners all the time and destroy them without our knowledge. In fact, when you find an enlarged lymph node, chances are you've found an active POW camp during its questioning period. Holding prisoners for questioning is a crucial step: lymph nodes need to know who these cells are before they can destroy them. At this time nodes will feel very small and hard, but after a menstrual cycle or two, they will just disappear; sometimes, these little nodes might even feel tender to the touch. The bottom line is this: small lumps that go away after two or three cycles are never cancerous. They are normal, healthy lymph nodes doing their job.

Enlarged lymph nodes that **don't** *disappear (are suspicious)*

These are usually found on the neck area or under the arm, but they can occur in the breast as well. When your lymph nodes are invaded by malignant cells, the cancer is in a later stage—it would have been around for a long time to have progressed to the lymph nodes. Here, the lymph nodes try to "question" and destroy the cells, but since the cells are so primitive, the lymph nodes become confused and hold the cells indefinitely, which is why the nodes remain enlarged. It is unlikely that you'll feel these kind of nodes in your breast—most often, you'll feel them under your arm—but the malignant cells would have originated from your breast. If you feel an enlarged lymph node under your arm or on your breast, you'll need to get it investigated. Generally, if it disappears after one or two cycles, it's nothing to worry about. If it doesn't go away, further tests and biopsies are called for. If you feel an enlarged node around your collar bone, get it checked immediately—it's too far from your breast to be affected by menstrual cycle changes.

The suspicious lump

A suspicious lump is usually hard and painless, but cancerous lumps have been known to be painful as well. The most important characteristic about a suspicious lump is that it tends to remain unchanged at your next cycle, if you're menstruating—breasts can change drastically from one cycle to the next, and sometimes the lumps disappear. Unchanged means that the lump stays in the same place in your breast and doesn't suddenly hurt or shrink. (If it grows, you should be suspicious.) If you're past menopause, the lump won't be affected by cycle changes unless you're on hormone replacement therapy and must be investigated since women past menopause are in a higher risk group for breast cancer.

If the lump is painful, it may signify one of the benign breast conditions described earlier. If the lump shrinks or disappears in one cycle, then magically reappears the next, it is unlikely that it is cancerous and may just be part of normal breast "lumpiness." If the lump is smaller than half an inch, painless, and remains unchanged, it may be an enlarged lymph node, which you should have investigated.

If your lump is suspicious, don't panic. It is probably not cancer; more likely it is either a cyst (a benign lump filled with fluid); or a fibroadenoma (lazy benign cells living in a harmless clump); or a "pseudolump" (suspicious at first, but there for a good reason when investigated); or a a normal lymph node that has enlarged for harmless reasons.

Is a small lump "baby breast cancer?"

It is logical to think that breast cancer starts out as a small lump that just gets bigger as the cancer advances. But this is not so. Sometimes, a malignant lump develops because your body is reacting to cancerous cells. The body grows fibrous, scarlike tissue around the cancer cells, which makes the lump palpable ("feelable") to human touch. But don't count on this happening. Not all cancer that's palpable has this scar tissue around it.

What do I do when I feel a lump?

Whether or not you're still menstruating, get the lump looked at ASAP. Don't wait. Waiting will just create more anxiety. Although most breast cancer grows pretty slowly, it is important to be aggressive about diagnosing it and ruling out a malignancy. At the same time, it's important not to panic. In order for the lump to have formed, the cancer must have been growing for several years at least. Early breast cancer detected on a mammogram has generally been growing for about five to seven years; by the time a lump you can feel develops, the cancer has been around a long time. It is important to note, however, that the size of your breast lump has no relationship to the stage of cancer. In other words, a large lump doesn't necessarily mean you have a more advanced stage cancer, while a small lump doesn't necessarily mean you have an early stage cancer.

Why do breasts sprout "normal" lumps to begin with?

All women will find lumps in their breasts from time to time. Just like other parts of the body, breasts will change in size and shape as you age, diet, gain weight, and go from cycle to cycle. Large-breasted women may be plagued by lumpiness or nodules (small knots of usually benign cells) more frequently than small-breasted women. If you imagine the grape cluster again, some grapes in the cluster respond more to hormones than others. And that's where the lump comes from.

INVESTIGATING SUSPICIOUS BREAST LUMPS

When you discover your lump, don't wait to see if it disappears on its own. Breast specialists recommend that you arrange to see a breast specialist for your suspicious breast lump right away; your primary care doctor can refer you to one. If you live in an area where there are no breast specialists, you may want to consider going to a larger center.

Ultimately, whoever handles the investigation must first take a medical history to assess your risk of breast cancer in the first place and do a thorough breast exam. The second step is to have a either a mammogram or an ultrasound. An ultrasound will tell your doctor whether the lump in your breast is solid or filled with fluid—the presence of fluid means it's a cyst. The imaging test you have depends on your age. If you're under thirty, for example, most doctors would probably want to first do an ultrasound and only move on to a mammogram if further tests were required.

A needle aspiration procedure (see figure 2.4) may be done after your imaging test. This is a simple in-office procedure performed under a local anesthetic. A long needle is used to suck out any fluid from the lump. This will immediately tell the doctor whether the lump is a cyst (a fluid-filled lump), which is usually harmless.

However, it is very important that you have your imaging test before a needle is inserted into your lump. That's because there may be some bleeding from the needle aspiration procedure, which can make interpretation of your imaging test more difficult.

Cysts

Usually, a lump filled with fluid of any kind (often milk if you're lactating) is a cyst and is not cancerous at all. Most cysts are benign. If your cyst is discovered via an ultrasound, your doctor may choose not to bother sucking out the fluid unless the cyst is bothering you. If the doctor is performing a needle aspiration, the cyst will collapse or deflate when the fluid is sucked out. Then, no more lump. If blood comes out with the fluid, the cells will be sent to a pathologist for examination, but this may not be a sign of cancer, just of a possible infection.

Figure 2.3
DEEP AND SHALLOW CYSTS

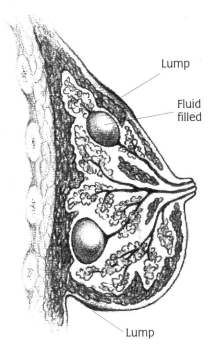

Lump

Fluid
filled

Lump

Figure 2.4
ASPIRATING A CYST

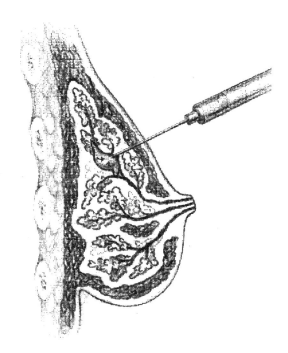

There is a 1 percent chance that your cyst may contain cancerous cells called intracystic papillary carcinoma. Like the papillary carcinoma discussed in the next chapter, here the cancer is restricted only to the cyst (hence the word *intracystic*) and does not spread beyond it. If this is the case, the cyst will also be removed.

A collapsed cyst can sometimes come back. If this happens, you may want to have a lumpectomy. If the lump doesn't go down after the fluid is removed from the cyst, your doctor may want to do a cellular biopsy procedure known as fine-needle aspiration. This is similar to the needle aspiration procedure, but involves sucking out the cells from the lump. The cells are then sent to a laboratory for further investigation.

Figure 2.5
FIBROADENDOMA

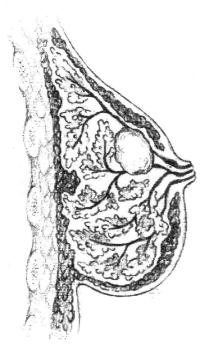

Sometimes, no fluid will come out of the cyst your doctor is trying to aspirate (suck out). At this point, a cellular biopsy may also be done as a double check. (Indeed, sometimes doctors miss the fluid if they aspirate from a strange angle.) Cysts are most common in women approaching menopause (women in their late forties and early fifties), but can occur when you're in your thirties and forties or younger. It is also common for women to develop numerous cysts or recurring cysts.

Fibroadenomas

This is a very common solid benign lump (shown in figure 2.5). It evolves when you cross an adenoma (a clump of benign glandular cells—the breast has loads of glands within it) with a fibroma (a clump of benign cells made out of connective tissue in the breast). If your lump isn't a cyst, chances are it is an adenoma or a fibroma.

A fibroadenoma feels like a marble inside your breast and is often very close to the nipple. Sometimes it can be the size of an egg, in which case it is known as a giant fibroadenoma. Actually, a fibroadenoma is a kind of "breast fibroid," a harmless overgrowth of normal breast tissue. (You don't have to have a uterine fibroid to have a breast fibroid or vice versa, nor does one kind of fibroid predispose you to the other.)

Fibroadenomas are suspected when the lump turns out to be solid at an ultrasound or when no fluid comes out when it is aspirated by a needle. The diagnosis is confirmed by two biopsy procedures. The first is a fine-needle aspiration, described earlier. If the cellular examination comes back negative, it means that there is likely no cancer, but the doctor may proceed with a surgical biopsy. This is really a lumpectomy, in which the lump is surgically removed at a hospital under a local or general anesthetic.

Doctors can usually tell the difference between a fibroadenoma and a malignant lump just by feeling it with their fingers, but some may take out the lump anyway so you won't confuse future new lumps with it. The biopsy may also give the doctor an opportunity to examine all parts of the lump to ensure that nothing has been missed.

Many breast centers, however, are re-evaluating the need to automatically remove fibroadenomas (which are confirmed by an examination of the cells or the tissue obtained from a core needle biopsy) in women under age thirty. Fibroadenomas are most common in younger women in their teens and twenties, but they're seen in older women, too. Like cysts, recurring (or even several) fibroadenomas are common.

"Pseudolumps"

This is a term coined by Susan Love, M.D., and refers to the "oops—I didnt realize this is supposed to be here" category of bumps. They look and feel like lumps, but then turn out to be "extra lumpy" breast tissue that in fact has every right to be there. This extra lumpy tissue can result from either dead fat tissue lying around from a previous biopsy; or hardened scar tissue from past breast surgery; or hardened silicone from an implant; or the kind of lump that forms in fibrocystic breast condition (discussed later).

In summary, it is sometimes difficult for doctors to distinguish suspicious breast lumps from non-suspicious lumps. An experienced breast specialist will take a thorough medical history, do a physical exam and a high quality mammogram and/or ultrasound, and will try to aspirate the lump. Then, based on the results of your exam, history, and tests, the doctor will decide whether the lump needs to come out.

Enlarged lymph nodes

Enlarged lymph nodes that don't go away (see earlier discussion) are treated like other lumps by needle aspiration, followed by fine-needle aspiration, followed by lumpectomy. Enlarged lymph nodes are usually found under the arm and will be investigated for evidence of a metastasis, the spreading of malignant cells. Lymph nodes often enlarge for unknown reasons, however, and are not cancerous. (A nasty virus can render a lymph node permanently enlarged, for example.) If the lump is solid but going to be removed anyway, why bother with a fine-needle aspiration at all? A fine-needle aspiration tells the doctor whether the cells inside the lump are cancerous. In fact, this biopsy is more accurate in detecting a malignant condition than a benign one. It is done more as a "ruling out" procedure than anything else. If your result is positive, it means that the lump is malignant. This helps the physician plan the next step: a wide excision surgery as part of a breast conservation to try to obtain clear margins (see Chapter 3, page 113). But even if the doctor suspects the lump is benign and the fine-needle aspiration comes out negative, the doctor may still not know for sure. Taking the lump out immediately is best; it avoids future lump "confusion," too. Breast cancer is discussed in the next chapter.

SCREENING FOR BREAST CANCER AND SUSPICIOUS LUMPS

Most breast lumps are not cancerous. Although knowing your family history and your risks is an important part of breast cancer awareness (see Chapter 1), it's also important to note that 70 percent of all breast cancer occurs in women with none of the known risk factors (discussed in Chapter 1, too). Breast cancer can only be detected from a suspicious lump in the breast—which is discovered either by you, or a doctor, or by mammography. So, mammography is used for two purposes: as a diagnostic tool for women who need to find the cause of various breast problems (lumps, pain, and so on) and as a screening tool to help detect early breast cancers in women who are not exhibiting any signs or symptoms of breast cancer. The controversy over mammography is its use as a screener, not as a diagnostic tool.

Depending on which set of guidelines you're following, many women will not have a mammography until they themselves feel a lump. And that can be a scary process. Other non-radiation-emitting methods have been explored (thermal screenings, heat sensors, and ultrasound have been used in the past), but nothing has come close to being as effective as mammography combined with breast self-exam (BSE). Generally, ultrasound is only helpful as a diagnostic tool for a specific lump that has been found, but doesn't help to locate new ones.

For the moment, mammography combined with a monthly BSE is still the most reliable screening method for breast cancer. An Israeli researcher reported in 1993 that she obtained the same screening results with Magnetic Resonance Imaging (MRI) as she did with mammography. MRI has the benefit of having no radiation, which is promising, but needs to be researched further before North American hospitals will consider it more accurate than mammography. Moreover, MRI is not useful in finding calcification, which is often an initial finding of breast cancer on a mammogram, and is really expensive, making it unaffordable for many hospitals. In Canada, for example, many major cities are lucky if they have one MRI machine.

Finally, a better screening method is being explored—genetic screening. These are blood tests that can detect the breast cancer genes BRCA1 and BRCA2, discussed in Chapter 1. Research is also underway to develop a "cancer chip" using information technology. The chip would be able to detect cancer within a cell's DNA from a simple blood sample.

Currently, there is a blood test known as the CA 15-3 which detects tiny "sloughed off" cells produced by malignant tumors in the bloodstream. This is only used to detect breast cancer recurrence, however, and its effectiveness as a screening method for even that is still being debated.

BSE: BREAST SELF-EXAMINATION

This method should be called "get to know your breasts." It is shown in figure 2.7 on pages 69 and 70. It involves feeling your breasts in a specific way at the same time each month and distinguishing suspicious lumps from normal lumps and bumps. You can't know if a lump has remained "unchanged" unless you've been checking your breasts every month. While ideally, you should begin BSE by age twenty, starting at any age is fine.

If you haven't reached menopause, you'll need to do a BSE after each period ends, when your breasts are least tender and lumpy. When you're pregnant, a BSE should be done every month. When you're breastfeeding, do a monthly

Figure 2.6
PEAU D'ORANGE

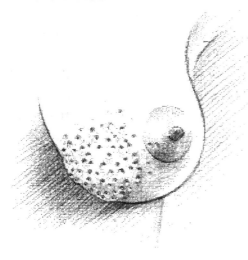

BSE after a feeding, when your breasts aren't filled with milk. (After your periods return, perform BSEs after a feeding, and after your period is over.) If you're past menopause, just pick the same time each month to do it.

Although the steps to BSE are outlined in the following section, make sure your doctor actually shows you how to do it as well. In addition, there is a kit available through the National Cancer Institute (listed at the back of this book) called the *Mammacare Learning System*, which consists of a 45-minute video and a 30-page instructional manual. The kit is designed to teach you how to do a breast self-exam using what's known as a vertical grid pattern, currently the most effective pattern. The kit was developed at the University of Florida and was partially funded by the National Cancer Institute.

At any rate, here are the steps of a BSE:

1. *Visually inspect your breasts.* Stand in front of the mirror and look closely at your breasts. You're looking for *peau d'orange*—dimpling, puckering (like an orange peel)—and noticeable lumps. Do you see any discharge that dribbles out on its own or any bleeding from the nipple? Any funny dry patches on the nipple (which may be Paget's disease)?

2. *Visually inspect your breasts with your arms raised.* Now, raise your arms over your head in front of the mirror and look for the same thing: dimpling, puckering, and noticeable lumps. Raising your arms smoothes out the breast a little more so these changes are more obvious.

3. *Palpate (feel your breast).* Lie down on your bed with a pillow under your left shoulder and place your left hand under your head. With the flat part of the fingertips of your right hand, examine your left breast for a

Figure 2.7
BREAST SELF-EXAMINATION

1.

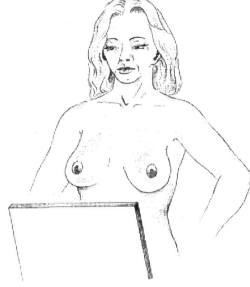

Look for visual changes

2.

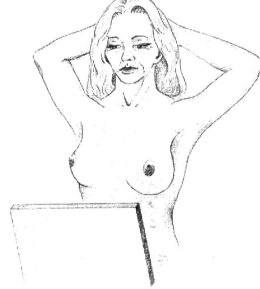

Repeat with arms raised

3.

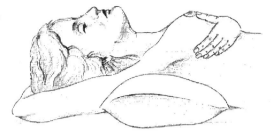

Feel the breast in a circular motion

4.

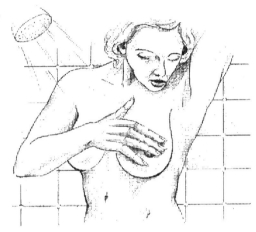

You can do this in the shower . . .

5.

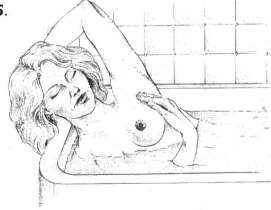

or while in the bathtub

Figure 2.7 *continued*
BREAST SELF-EXAMINATION

1.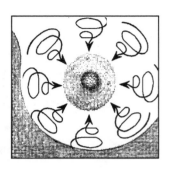

2.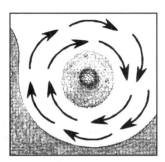

3.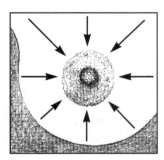

4.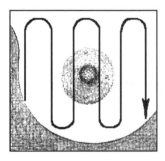

Pick one of the patterns shown above as your palpation "route" for your BSE.

lump, using a gentle circular motion. Imagine that the breast is a clock, and make sure you feel each hour, as well as the nipple area and armpit area.

4. *Repeat step 3, but reverse sides, examining your right breast with your left hand.*

5. *If you find a lump.* Note the size and shape of any lump you find and see how painful it is. A lump that should cause suspicion is usually painless, is about one-fourth inch to a half inch in size and remains unchanged from month to month. Get your lump looked at as soon as you can, or if you're comfortable waiting, hold on until the next cycle/month. If the lump changes in the next cycle by shrinking or becoming painful, it's not cancerous, but get it looked at anyway. If the suspicious lump stays the same, get it checked as soon as possible. Keep in mind that breast cysts are common, variable in size, and occasionally tender.

   6. *If discharge oozes out of your nipple on its own or if blood comes out, see your doctor immediately.* Don't wait.

   7. *If your nipple is dry and patchy, see your doctor immediately.* Don't wait.

How effective is a manual breast exam?

Two-thirds of all breast cancers are discovered by women themselves—either accidentally or through a BSE. Although you should have a clinical breast exam (where your doctor manually feels your breasts for abnormalities) done with your annual Pap tests, too, not all doctors are experts in doing clinical breast exams. That's why doing a BSE yourself is an extremely important screening method. BSEs are also important in areas where doctors or routine mammography are not widely available.

Studies that examined the effect of BSE on tumor size have found that BSEs enable women to find smaller tumors than they would find accidentally. Surprisingly, though, primary care physicians may pick up about only one cancer every five years by doing a clinical breast exam. The moral here: God helps those who help themselves!

THE INCREDIBLE ADVENTURES OF MAMMOGRAPHY GUIDELINES

Depending on what you read and which experts you talk to, you will hear two sets of mammography screening guidelines: "mammography at fifty" and "mammography at forty."

Well, there are valid arguments for either set of guidelines, but many women are alive today because they had a routine mammogram before they were fifty. Nevertheless, I've boiled down the arguments for both sides.

Argument for "mammography at fifty" (routine screening to begin at age fifty)

Advocates in this camp will point to the fact that breast cancer incidence rises after age fifty (i.e., after menopause). But, the truth is, the rate of increased risk is actually highest *until* age fifty and drops slightly after that.

Another theory is that premenopausal breast tissue is less fatty and more dense and therefore more difficult to compress, to read, and to interpret. Thus, the younger the woman, the less fatty the breast tissue, and hence, the harder her mammogram it is to read and interpret. The older the woman, the easier it is to read and interpret the mammogram.

Critics of mammography at forty also wonder if the radiation delivered to breast tissue when mammography is done on women younger than age fifty is actually responsible for the increase in breast cancer after fifty. But supporters of mammography at forty say this claim is not logical, considering that the equipment used today delivers far less radiation than it did even five years ago, and point to the fact that there are no studies that support the claim.

Another argument involves the false positive rate of mammography. Abnormalities found on mammograms often turn out to be a cyst or a fibroadenoma that is not cancerous. Only one-fifth of all abnormalities found on mammograms turn out to be malignant and the rate of false positives is higher in younger women. In the United States, only 20 to 30 percent of the roughly 600,000 breast biopsies done per year for mammographic abnormalities are actually malignant. Therefore 580,000 women will go through the emotional rollercoaster of having breast biopsies for no reason. In fact, the emotional toll of being told a mammogram is positive has actually been costed out and found to be a significant sum. (Two recent suicides in Britain were reportedly linked to positive mammogram results.) Should younger women be subjected to the emotional stress of a false positive? Or, should younger women risk having a breast cancer missed because they followed the "at fifty" guideline? Breast cancer activists have also raised the touchy issue of profit: The younger the age at which breast cancer screening begins, the more money somebody is making. Roughly 51.5 million women in the United States alone are over 40. When you factor in how much a mammogram costs per woman ($50-$250 in the U.S.), you get rather large profits.

And finally, there are no conclusive studies showing a benefit of mammography prior to age fifty (that is, screening does not significantly lower mortality from breast cancer). The problem has a lot to do with how statisticians add up the benefits. Let's say an invasive tumor is growing inside you, which will kill you in five years—regardless of whether you discover the cancer today from a mammogram (which can find a tumor as early as two years before it can be felt by hand) or two years from now through BSE. The "benefit" in this case is that you will spend the next two years with the knowledge that you have cancer, probably in treatment. After you die, a statistician will say that the mammogram lengthened your survival because the date of diagnosis was two years earlier than it would have been without that mammogram. With the mammogram, you lived with cancer for five years; without the mammogram, you lived with cancer for three years. This is what's called "lead time bias" which can essentially create a victory for medicine when none exists. In other words, you're still dead in five years, mammogram or not.

And then, there is the opposite scenario. A small in situ (non-invasive) breast tumor is growing inside you; if left alone, it will never pose a threat and you will live out a normal life. But instead, you have a mammogram, the tumor is found, you go through treatment and distress. Prior to mammography, only 1 to 2 percent of all breast cancers were in situ tumors; today 10 percent of all breast cancers are in situ tumors. Is mammography finding deadly cancer earlier or just finding more tumors, many of which are not harmful?

Argument for "mammography at forty" (routine screening to begin at age forty)

Advocates in this camp maintain that since the studies regarding the screening age for mammography are debatable, and since the rate of increased risk is highest until age fifty, it makes sense to screen women as early as possible. About 18 percent of all breast cancers occur in 40-something women, and twice as many women under 40 are diagnosed with breast cancer today than in 1970. Furthermore, breast cancers can behave in different ways; some grow faster than others. So there is always a risk of someone falling between the cracks if we recommend screening at an older age.

A new theory about the nature of breast cancer supports mammography at 40 more than ever. According to a *New York Times* report, some experts believe that there are three different types of breast cancer: one type grows and spreads very quickly, within a matter of months, while the second type takes between five and ten years to grow. And the third type takes longer than five to ten years to grow. It's believed that this is the reason why studies have trouble showing a clear benefit to mammography at 40 versus 50.

The study most quoted for showing the benefits of mammography at forty is the HIP study. This 1963 study looked at 62,000 women aged forty to sixty-four who were enrolled in New York's Health Insurance Plan (HIP). Both a control and a test group were set up to evaluate the benefits of mammography. Women in the test group had a physical exam and a mammogram every year for five years. Women in the control group had no special treatment. Ten years later, breast cancer deaths in the test group were down by 30 percent. A more recent analysis, published in the journal *Cancer*, concludes that annual mammograms do indeed reduce cancer deaths in women under 50.

Critics of the study, however, argue that it never specified the optimum *age* for a mammogram. They also believe that screening at forty will lead to routine screening of younger and younger women, which would prove to be of no benefit and, because of radiation, could actually be damaging.

Who recommends what?

The American College of Obstetricians and Gynecologists, the American College of Radiologists, and their Canadian, British, Swedish, Dutch, and Italian counterparts recommend annual mammographies for women age fifty or older. The American College of Physicians recommends mammograms every two years for women age fifty or older. In this age group, routine mammography (every two to three years) seems to reduce annual mortality rates by 20 to 40 percent.

The American Medical Association, The National Cancer Institute, and The American Cancer Society *were* recommending screenings every one or two years for women forty years and older; but in light of a 1992 Canadian study (which many experts dismissed as flawed), guidelines went into flux, and seemed to revert back to screening at 50, although the American Cancer Society continued to recommend screening at 40.

The most recent twist occurred in 1997, when a 13-member panel of doctors, statisticians, academic researchers, lay people, and activists, met for three days at the National Institutes of Health to settle the guideline debate once and for all. They couldn't. Their recommendation was that women in their 40s must decide for themselves. The American Cancer Society and The National Cancer Institute disapproved of this vague recommendation, which causes even more confusion. Right now, The American Cancer Society recommends that women in their 40s be screened, and that women 50 and older should have annual mammograms. The 13-member panel did agree that if younger women were to be screened, screening should be done annually since tumors grow faster in this age group.

What should you do?

You have to make your screening decision based on your level of personal comfort. Since the density of your breasts will change radically after menopause, having, as the American Medical Association recommends, a baseline mammogram sometime between thirty-five and thirty-nine (which in theory, can be compared to future mammograms) is probably not very useful because it is like comparing melons to apples. However, a baseline mammogram can pick up abnormalities.

Obviously, the guidelines for mammography are conflicting. So here are some other guidelines to use in deciding what to do about mammography:

- Any time you find a suspicious lump, a mammogram will help to determine what's going on. No matter how old you are, or what your risk factors are, have a mammography. Period. If there's a question about your screening center's credibility (by word of mouth, for example, or a bad experience you had), get a second one done at another center.

- If you have any family history of estrogen-dependent cancers, such as breast cancer, ovarian cancer, or colon cancer, earlier routine screening (starting at age forty) may be a good idea and can offer you some comfort. Many experts recommend an annual screening after age forty with this kind of family history. If your mother, sister, or grandmother had breast cancer, you may even want to consider mammography at age thirty-five.

- Anyone else who faces the many questionable risks raised in Chapter 1, and is concerned, can make some lifestyle and dietary adjustments discussed in Chapter 10 (although this is not a recipe for prevention). Then, beginning routine screening at the guideline age you're comfortable with makes the most sense.

- Regardless of your age, you should be doing BSEs and familiarizing yourself with your breasts so you will notice anything unusual. You should also make sure that a manual breast exam is performed by your doctor each year along with your Pap smears.

MAXIMIZING MAMMOGRAPHY

The screening guidelines for mammography may remain in conflict, but mammography is still the only reliable imaging test available as of this writing. Other techniques such as the sensitive ultrasound screening and MRI imaging are still being debated, so, for now, outside of feeling your own breast regularly, you have to make the best of mammography, which currently carries between a 10 to 15 percent false negative rate and a much higher false positive rate. Newer imaging techniques may help to improve a mammogram's accuracy, such as injectable "tracers," digital technology, and technologies once designed for military defense.

As shown in figure 2.8, a mammogram is a breast X ray. It is used as both a routine screening procedure for breast cancer (see Chapter 1), as well as a diagnostic tool to investigate suspicious lumps. It is similar to a chest X ray except it is limited to just the breast and does not display the lungs. Mammography involves sticking your breast inside a machine with a plastic plate that is covered with another metal plate. A picture is then taken of the breast. If an abnormality is found, an ultrasound is usually done.

Common fears

Many women avoid even routine mammography after age fifty either because they fear pain and radiation or because they fear the possibility of a positive result. Other barriers to mammography include a lack of education about when and why to have one, lack of transportation to a screening center, language difficulties, cultural issues, and even illiteracy. Clearly, it is impossible for all these barriers to be removed, but if you have a relative or friend, for example, who refuses to have a mammogram because of some of these reasons, you can help to educate her by translating or explaining information that you receive or by accompanying her to a physician (hers or yours) who can help explain screening to her. In fact, the sex of a woman's physician often has a lot to do with screening behavior, particularly in the senior population. More women are likely to have the appropriate screening done if their physician is female.

How to get the most out of your mammogram

1. Go to a reliable screening center, one that specializes in mammograms and does at least twenty to thirty mammograms per day. In the United States, look for an accredited ACR (American College of Radiologists) mammography center, or call 1-800-4-CANCER for an FDA-certified center.

2. The X ray image of the breast must be of the highest quality. Good equipment that is used only for mammography and has been purchased no later than three years ago is your best bet. Cheap or older equipment used by a cut-rate center will be of no value to you—and it could deliver false positives.

3. A dedicated, experienced technician specially trained in mammography must perform the screening. Ideally, you should ask if the radiologist interpreting your mammogram specializes in breast radiology (this is not very common). Some specialists recommend that at least two experienced radiologists read and interpret mammogram results, but this is expensive, and if the two radiologists reading the mammogram do not

Figure 2.8
MAMMOGRAPHY PROCEDURE

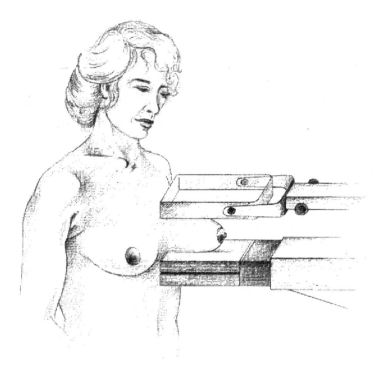

specialize in mammography, you're probably no further ahead. So, ask your mammogram facility questions such as how many mammograms the radiologist has read and what the facility's "call-back" record is (that is, how many second looks does the facility do). A reasonable number is 10 percent or less. A high call-back rate is suspicious because it suggests that the radiologist may be insecure about the readings and keeps rechecking for tiny little things. If the facility doesn't know the call-back record, go elsewhere; it's a sign that it does not have very good quality control.

4. For the mammogram to be as accurate as possible, the breast must be compressed as much as possible (so it may hurt a little bit). Compression also reduces the amount of radiation required. Experts suggest going for a

mammogram after your period, when your breasts are least tender. You can also take an over-the-counter painkiller an hour before the test.

5. How much time is spent per patient in the mammography room? Anything less than twenty minutes per patient is too fast.

6. The center should have a strict quality-control program in place. Ask the facility to show you their quality assurance data. A good statistic for a facility is roughly 20 to 40 percent of cancers out of a hundred biopsies. If it is less than that, the facility is probably "overbiopsing"; and if it is higher, they are too lax and may be missing cancers. All reliable facilities should be able to show you their quality assurance data. Ask about what the facility does to ensure quality before you have the procedure. If it does not have such a program, find another center.

7. A physical examination of the breasts by a trained nurse or qualified physician must accompany the mammogram. Before you have the mammogram, however, you may want to see your doctor, who will address any concerns he or she has on your mammogram requisition. In fact, the best facilities have one radiologist do the clinical exam, read the mammogram, and perform an ultrasound. That way, when it is time to interpret the mammogram, the radiologist has all the information components needed to interpret it as accurately as possible.

8. Don't wear any talcum powder, deodorant, or lotions on your upper body the day you're scheduled for your mammogram. Little flecks of these products can get on the plates and interfere with the results.

Interpreting results

Ten radiologists can have ten different interpretations of one mammography and ten different recommendations of "what to do next." Variations in mammogram interpretations have to do with many factors, including

1. *Visual observations.* One radiologist can see a lesion in a given film, another may miss it altogether.

2. *Perception.* One tumor (a.k.a. "mass") may be perceived as "probably

benign" by Radiologist A and "probably cancerous" by Radiologist B. It's the same principle as the half-full—half-empty glass. It all depends on your personality and perspective.

3. *Concern.* Some radiologists will follow up every observed abnormality—no matter how small—with further tests, while others may reserve follow-up tests for "highly suspicious" abnormalities. Again, this depends on the personality of the radiologist looking at the film.

4. *Variables.* Your age, the size of your breasts, your medical history, and the quality of the mammography equipment are all variables.

Current studies show that mammogram interpretations vary so much that some patients with cancer were not identified. In fact, almost 30 percent of the cancers in a 1987 study were incorrectly categorized when the films were originally interpreted. Many experts currently recommend that since radiologists differ in what they catch or miss, two observers for one mammogram is the best route, but other experts point out that one mammographer specializing solely in breast radiology may still be better than two who are not specialists. For what it's worth, in Sweden, whose mammography interpretation and standards are considered the best in the world, having two radiologists examine every mammogram has increased the cancer detection rate by 15 percent.

· · · · · · ·

I hope I have answered the "is it or isn't it cancer" question. If you do hear the dreaded "it is cancer," Chapter 3 is the one to read. Not only do I explain in non-technical terms exactly what cancer is and what kinds of cancer there are, but I discuss all other questions, options, and choices you might have. As well, treatment issues, side effects, and success/failure rates are explored in detail.

CHAPTER 3
· · · · · · ·

WHEN THEY SAY IT'S MALIGNANT

This chapter will take you through the journey of first being diagnosed with breast cancer. It provides a non-technical explanation of what cancer actually is and the various types of breast cancer women are diagnosed with. It also explains the various stages of breast cancer and the system doctors use to tell what stage the cancer is in.

A detailed section on dealing with diagnosis and doctors will give you important guidelines for asking questions about your cancer, educating yourself about your particular diagnosis, and deciding how to discuss your condition with friends and family members.

This chapter then explains the current treatment philosophies: local therapy, systemic therapy, and adjuvant therapy. All three involve a different approach to breast cancer, mean different sacrifices and different consequences for every woman, and will therefore require every woman to make her own decision.

Finally, this chapter sees you through your surgery. No matter what stage your cancer is in, some form of surgery will probably be recommended (although you do have the right to refuse it), be it a lumpectomy (removal of a breast tumor) or a mastectomy (removal of the breast). Treatments following surgery such as radiation, chemotherapy, and hormone therapy are discussed in detail in Chapter 4. Alternative medicine is discussed in Chapter 7, and breast reconstruction and breast implants are discussed in Chapter 5.

Being diagnosed with any kind of cancer is like landing in a foreign country. You are suddenly faced with all kinds of barriers: language barriers, in the sense that everything is in medicalspeak; cultural barriers, in the sense that hospital life doesn't work like other environments you are used to; and a lack of friends, in the sense that you suddenly feel isolated and are surrounded by strangers. So, cancer patients usually go through a crash course on their particular kind of cancer. They get educated, they learn how to navigate and maximize hospital visits, and they ultimately discover parts of themselves they never knew existed. Let's get started, so you can get on with treatment decisions and the rest of your life.

WHAT IS CANCER?

Cancer is the general term for abnormal growth of cells—a cluster of cells that go out of control and multiply. When the abnormal cell reproduces, it has the ability to invade, or metastasize to, other parts of the body. The word *cancer* is Latin for crab. It was, in fact, the crab-like appearance of advanced breast tumors that inspired the Roman physician Galen to actually name cancer crab, but the Greek word *karkinos* originally meant crab, too, which is how Hippocrates first identified and classified this illness 2,500 years ago.

Cancer was an extremely rare disease in the ancient world and is not mentioned at all in the Bible or the *Yellow Emperor's Classic of Internal Medicine,* the ancient medicine book of China. It began to be seen more extensively around the time of the Industrial Revolution, and by the start of this century, the annual mortality rate from cancer in the United States was about 4 percent.

Actually, the cancer cell itself is not dangerous (unlike bacterias or viruses), but its impact on the rest of your organs is. As cancer cells spread into various parts of your body, they interfere with the jobs of regular cells, confuse other organs, and can wreak havoc on your body. A cancer cell is basically a terrorist cell that hijacks organs and other cells. Cancer cells use the lymph system to get into the bloodstream and then travel throughout the body. These cells love organs that have multiple blood vessels and nutrients; organs such as bones, lungs, and the brain are common areas where cancer spreads.

LEARNING THE LANGUAGE

Cancer cells are divided into two groups: carcinoma and sarcoma. A carcinoma refers to cancerous cells made of epithelial cells, which are cells that line various tissues. You'll find carcinomas in organs that tend to secrete some fluid (milk, mucus, digestive juices, and so on). Common sites for carcinomas are breasts, lungs, and the colon; common gynecological sites are the ovaries, cervix, and the endometrium. Carcinomas account for 80 to 90 percent of all human cancers. They are generally slow-growing. The prefix that is always attached to the word *carcinoma* will tell you where the carcinoma is growing and the kind of cells that are involved. An adenocarcinoma, for example, is a carcinoma made of glandular cells. Carcinoma cells can be benign or malignant. The word *oma* by itself means benign. An adenoma refers to a clump of benign glandular cells, a fibroma refers to a clump of benign fibrous cells, and so on. When the cells are malignant, the word *carcinoma* is attached to the end, as in adenocarcinoma. If your breast cancer is referred to as an adenocarcinoma, this tells you that your cancer originated in glandular tissue. It gets even more specific. You'll need to know exactly where the adenocarcinoma itself originated. You may be told, for example, that you have either a ductal carcinoma or lobular carcinoma, which means that your adenocarcinoma originated in either the breast ducts or lobes, especially. Since both ducts and lobes are a kind of gland, malignant cells that develop here will always be adenocarcinomas.

Think of it like this: using the word *carcinoma* by itself is as descriptive as saying sweater. Adenocarcinoma is like saying wool sweater. A more specific description such as ductal adenocarcinoma is like saying lambswool sweater or angora sweater. And there can be other prefixes that are synonymous with saying blue angora sweater. Papillary ductal carcinoma describes the shape of the cancer cell, and would be like saying V-necked, angora sweater, and so on. The point being that you need not worry about a lengthy, unpronounceable name that may be attached to your cancer; if a long prefix is attached to the word *carcinoma,* it is just describing it more accurately. There are literally hundreds of carcinomas, all described by a different combination of prefixes that identify the part of the body that is involved, the shape of the carcinoma, etc. Like many diseases, carcinomas are sometimes named after the doctor who discovered them. Paget's disease, a kind of breast skin cancer, is an example of this.

Sarcomas are cancerous cells made up of supporting connective tissue, such as the uterus. Sarcomas are rare and account for only 2 percent of all human cancers but tend to be more aggressive than carcinomas. Again, the prefixes before the word tell you where the sarcoma is located, what it is made of, what shape it is, etc. Sometimes sarcomas, too, are named after the doctors who discovered them.

The difference between a carcinoma and a sarcoma is the difference between a sweater and a boot; both have different physical properties, but are related. (You can also have a carcinosarcoma—a carcinoma and sarcoma all in one.)

In situ versus invasive

Regardless of whether you have a carcinoma or a sarcoma of some kind, the most important words are these: *in situ* and *invasive.* In situ means "in one place." A carcinoma in situ is confined to a specific area and has not spread. This is good news—it means that your cancer is, by definition, non-invasive, and is in an early stage. As discussed in the last chapter, mammography is finding many more in situ tumors. As a result, the incidence of in situ tumors has increased five to ten times. Twenty years ago, only 1 to 2 percent of all breast tumors were in situ; today 10 percent of all breast tumors are in situ. Invasive carcinoma is a carcinoma that has spread to local tissues, surrounding tissues, lymph nodes, or other organs. This is not good news, of course: it means that your cancer is in a later stage. But even though a cancer is invasive and at a later stage, such as a stage 1B breast cancer with a tumor size of 5 to 10 mm, for example, you still have a greater than 90 percent chance of living for at least twenty years.

A word about microinvasion

Sometimes pathologists will diagnose an in situ cancer as having microinvasion. Well, if in situ means non-invasive, how can it be microinvasive at the same time? This is a question that many breast surgeons are asking, too, because it is a somewhat paradoxical diagnosis. In fact, what many pathologists see as microinvasion could be caused by a variety of factors, including poor handling of the tissue biopsy, freezing, the way the tissue is cauterized, and so on. Surgeons suggest now that if you have a diagnosis of, say, "ductal carcinoma in situ with microinvasion," you should ask that your slides be sent for another opinion to a pathologist who specializes in breast pathology.

Differentiated versus undifferentiated

Cancer cells are classified into two behavioral categories: differentiated and undifferentiated. These terms refer to the sophistication of the cancer cells. Differentiated cancer cells resemble the cells of their origin. A differentiated cancer cell that originates in the breast ducts will look and act like a normal ductal cell. In fact, these cancer cells might actually assist other cells with routine functions. Because differentiated cells spend some of their time assisting the body, they spend less time reproducing, and therefore take a lot longer to metastasize, or spread, to other parts of the body. But both differentiated and undifferentiated are equally treatable, the key factors being tumor size and lymph node status. A purely differentiated cell is often hard to find—the cell may look as if it is only moderately abnormal. So, there are subclassifications: moderately differentiated, well differentiated, and poorly differentiated. These subclassifications are known as the cell's grading. A high grade means that the cell is immature, poorly differentiated, and therefore faster growing; a low-grade cancer cell is mature, well differentiated, slow growing, and less aggressive. (This is a terribly basic explanation of cell grading, which is actually based on far more complex criteria.)

Undifferentiated cancer is made up of very primitive cells that look wild and untamed and bear little or no resemblance to the cells of origin. They do not assist the body at all and are therefore able to spend all their time reproducing. This is dangerous because the cells can spread faster. There are cases, though, when undifferentiated cancer is not very aggressive, and the cells look more wild than they behave. This is often the situation in breast cancers.

These different cells also mix. When cells mix the aggressiveness of the disease is affected. For example, you can have mostly differentiated cells mixed in with a few undifferentiated cells, or vice versa. The cells that are in the majority affect the behavior of the cancer: mostly differentiated cells will slow down whatever undifferentiated cells exist, while mostly undifferentiated cells speed up whatever differentiated cells exist.

There are dozens of other traits of cancer cells that have a direct bearing on how well they respond to treatment. For example, in breast cancer, many cancer cells respond to either estrogen or progesterone and hence can be treated with hormone therapy in addition to other traditional treatments. Pathologists can tell a lot about the behavior of cancer cells: they can tell where the cells invaded surrounding tissue and break down the metastasis into vascular invasion (cancer within a blood vessel) or lymphatic invasion (cancer within lymphatic vessels or lymph nodes); they can estimate how fast the cell is reproducing; and they can tell whether there are any dead cancer cells around—if there are, it means that they are growing so fast that they have cut off their own blood supply and are leaving a trail of dead cells (called necrosis). All these factors are important and will affect your treatment and prognosis. Where the cancer is growing determines the kind of cancer cell you have. For example, breast cancer will spread as breast cancer cells, the cells won't suddenly turn into liver cancer cells when they reach your liver or become lymphoma as soon as they reach your lymph nodes. Ovarian cancer cells will continue to be ovarian cancer cells even in the abdomen, and so on.

DESIGNER GENES

As discussed in Chapter 1, we now know that genetics plays a role in a variety of cancers, particularly glandular cancers, such as breast cancer and ovarian cancer. That is why it is important for your doctor to know whether any cancers run in the family. Women whose mothers or sisters had breast cancer are more likely to develop it as well. This has prompted researchers to try to isolate specific oncogenes within our genetic makeup. The word *onco* means tumor; oncology is thus tumorology.

One theory is that every individual has certain oncogenes that remain dormant until an external agent switches them on. Once turned on, the oncogene transforms normal cells into abnormal cells. For example, if you carry the oncogene for breast cancer, many factors may trip its switch: poor diet, exposure to toxins, and so on. But what trips your switch may not trip your neighbor's breast cancer switch, which may be why some women get breast cancer and others do not. So in this sense, while cancers are believed to be genetic, external or environmental factors are believed to be responsible for triggering them.

Here's one way to think about it: we may all have some sort of weapon inside of us. Some of us have .38 caliber pistols, some of us have Uzis, some of us have cannons, and so on. But the hand that pulls the trigger only does so when it is repeatedly provoked by outside forces. In the case of breast cancer, tobacco, X rays, excess estrogen, sunlight, radioactive fallout, and industrial agents act as these provocative outside forces. So, while one cigarette may merely irritate your lung cells, twenty years of smoking may provide multiple hits to these cells that finally provokes them to pull the trigger.

Breast cancer is trickier to link to genetics because it is linked to a long list of other factors, chiefly estrogen. As discussed in previous chapters, breast cancer, uterine/endometrial cancer, and ovarian cancer are all estrogen-dependent, in that they are all linked to an increased amount of estrogen. Is the capacity to overproduce estrogen a genetic trait? Researchers believe this is a strong possibility.

All these factors make the future of cancer detection very promising. Blood tests that detect various oncogenes are already being developed, and by the year 2000, screening for a variety of oncogenes may be possible. This would mean that women can be treated or monitored long before the cancer becomes life-threatening.

Secondly, certain blood tests can now detect cancer trails (sheddings from cancer cells) in the bloodstream. The CA 15-3 blood test detects sheddings of breast cancer cells. This and other tests are currently being used to detect recurrences of breast cancer in women who have already received treatment.

Recurrence is discussed in Chapter 8. The role of genetics and cancer is also discussed in Chapter 1, page 20.

CANCER CULTURE

The adage "keep your friends close and your enemies closer" is very applicable when it comes to understanding cancer. You need to know the motives of cancer so you can grasp the motives of the various treatments you'll be offered.

Since cancer cells are living cells, it is in their nature to want to continue to live. So the first thing breast cancer cells do is grow—they'll simply begin growing where they first originated, be it a duct or a lobe. The next thing breast cancer cells do is change—they mutate from the other cells that surround it. After they get to a certain age, cancer cells want to move out and leave their original nest—this is when they spread out into surrounding fat and tissue.

A crucial motive of the cancer cell is eating. They do this by sending out protein messengers (called tumor angiogenesis factors) that create new blood vessels to feed it. If a cancer cell can manage these four basic functions—to grow, change, spread, and eat—it will live, which we experience as a tumor. If any of these functions are stopped, the cancer will die. Thus, treatment consists in interfering with at least one of these four functions: to stop the cells from growing; to stop the cells from changing or mutating; to stop the cells from spreading; or to stop the cells from eating.

If the cancer continues to live, it will simply continue these same basic behaviors: it will grow bigger; change and mutate even more to trick the immune system; and spread out even more by bursting into surrounding structures and into the blood vessels. Finally, if the cells reach adulthood, they want to settle down and find a good home, preferably an organ with a lining in its blood vessels like the liver, lungs, and bone. So the cells attach themselves to these blood vessels, and pass through it into the organ. The cells will continue to make themselves comfortable so they can reproduce more and more. This means setting themselves up with a new blood supply that will make the organ more conducive to their growth. And so it goes, until the cells occupy every space in the body. However, the most important thing to remember is that none of this happens immediately: it can take years for cancer cells to spread. So by the time you discover a lump, for example, the cancer may have already been around eight to ten years.

TYPES OF BREAST CANCER

There are several types of breast cancers one can develop; your type will be identified on your pathology report. The treatment route will depend greatly on what type of breast cancer you have. Most breast cancer is considered systemic, meaning that it involves the whole body, even if the tumor is localized. This is because it is assumed that on a microscopic level, other parts of the body may be involved at the time the tumor was discovered. Therefore, many women will be offered systemic treatment for a localized cancer (see the treatment section on page 111).

As discussed earlier, all cancers are initially classified as in situ (localized cancer that has not spread) or invasive (cancer that has spread), as well differentiated or undifferentiated. The following descriptions can have varying degrees of differentiation, and can be found in an in situ or invasive stage.

DUCTAL CARCINOMA (DUCTAL ADENOCARCINOMA)

It is estimated that 78 percent of all breast cancers fall into this category. Ductal carcinoma can be either invasive or noninvasive. Non-invasive ductal carcinoma is also called ductal carcinoma in situ (DCIS) or intraductal carcinoma. In fact, DCIS is an increasingly common cancer and accounts in some areas for 30 percent of all breast cancers. With the use of mammography becoming more widespread, experts estimate that one-third of all breast cancers will be DCIS by the year 2000. Treatment for this type of cancer varies greatly and depends on a whole batch of factors. In the past, the standard therapy for DCIS was surgery, followed by radiation, possibly followed by chemotherapy and/or hormone therapy (each discussed later). But today, treatment can range from lumpectomy to a bilateral mastectomy. If you are diagnosed with DCIS, you are urged to seek out at least two opinions from breast specialists regarding your treatment options.

Cell types

Breast cancer cells in the ducts come in different shapes and types. The shape determines how differentiated and, hence, aggressive the cancer is. About 75 percent of all ductal carcinomas do not have a specified shape. The rest come in about half a dozen distinct shapes; these ductal cancers have in fact been named after their shapes. Treatment will depend on how invasive the cancer is, regardless of shape.

Medullary carcinoma, which accounts for 1 to 4 percent of all invasive ductal breast cancers, is so named because the cancer is medulla-shaped or brain-shaped. This kind of breast cancer spreads fast and is made up of largely undifferentiated cells that spread through the lymphatic system. However, it generally has a better prognosis than other ductal cancers.

Colloid carcinoma accounts for about 1 to 3 percent of all invasive ductal breast cancers. In this type of cancer, the ducts are blocked with carcinoma cells, and cysts develop nearby. Staging will affect treatment, however.

Other types of ductal carcinoma include tubular, mucinous, scirrhous, and papillary (a finger-like pattern) carcinoma.

LOBULAR CARCINOMA

Representing about 9 to 15 percent of all breast cancers, lobular carcinoma can be invasive or non-invasive. Half of all lobular carcinomas are invasive and are known simply as lobular carcinoma. In terms of prognosis, staging, and treatment, invasive lobular carcinoma is the same as invasive ductal carcinoma, but lobular carcinoma has a specific appearance that gives it its name. In fact, experts believe that all breast cancers begin in the same place in the breast, and whether some grow into the lobule or stay within the duct is not important; what is important is that an invasive lobular cancer is not as easy to feel or see on a mammogram.

Treatment for invasive lobular carcinoma follows the same order as treatment for invasive ductal carcinoma: surgery (breast conserving or breast removal), possibly followed by radiation and/or chemotherapy.

The interesting thing about lobular carcinomas is that they are almost always estrogen-dependent, in that estrogen makes them grow, and can therefore be treated with hormone therapy. This is also the kind of cancer that is harder to find on a mammogram; it's not unusual for it to one day show up as a large cancer in women who have been having regular mammograms. Again, treatment depends on staging and what option you select.

LOBULAR CARCINOMA IN SITU (LCIS)

LCIS is actually not a cancer, not even a "premalignant" one, as you may have heard. It is really a marker that indicates you are at increased risk of developing invasive breast cancer at some future date. And women with LCIS may in fact develop invasive ductal carcinoma, as opposed to lobular. Basically, a diagnosis of LCIS means a red alert. You are officially at risk for developing invasive breast cancer in either one or both breasts, regardless of which side your LCIS was diagnosed. LCIS should never be confused with ductal carcinoma in situ, nor with invasive lobular carcinoma, discussed in the next paragraph. The treatment approach to LCIS is usually a watchful eye: a woman diagnosed with it should be having regular, high-quality mammograms and thorough clinical breast exams. Some women may be more comfortable having a prophylactic (preventive) mastectomy for this type of diagnosis. Prophylactic mastectomy is discussed in more detail in Chapter 10, which talks about prevention.

There are other types of breast cancer that develop atypically, such as Paget's disease or inflammatory breast cancer. These do not represent the majority of breast cancers. They also have rather atypical symptoms and treatments. Due to space restrictions, these cancers are not covered here. If you've been diagnosed with an atypical breast cancer, it is best to seek out very specific information from your surgeon and to do a literature search (see the resource section at the back of this book).

STAGING AND SPREADING

Four women can be diagnosed with the same kind of cancer, but it is quite possible that each of them will undergo completely different treatments and face a different prognosis. This happens because each of these women have a cancer that is at a different stage. To complicate matters even more, each cancer has its own "personality." So, the same type and stage of cancer may behave differently in different women. A cancer can be at any of four or five stages. Stage classification basically answers the question, where has it spread? Treatment and survival rates depend on what stage your cancer is in.

To detect what stage your cancer is in, you might have any of the following diagnostic tests: a chest X ray; another mammogram; various blood tests, including the CA 15-3, which is used to detect recurrence of a breast cancer or very advanced breast cancer but is not sensitive enough for early stage breast cancer, however; a CAT scan (computerized axial tomography), which takes pictures of your body in sections; and an MRI (magnetic resonance imaging), which helps to detect what is going on in the brain. Often a bone scan is done, in which radioactive particles are injected into your vein, then absorbed by bone, then picked up by a scanning machine, which will "count" how many radioactive particles remain in the bone. A high count is a sign that the bone needs to be X rayed further. Liver scans and an ultrasound may also be done.

As discussed earlier in this chapter, nearly all breast cancers are adenocarcinomas, that is, they originate in glandular tissue (the noted exceptions are inflammatory breast cancer and Paget's disease, which are both atypical). Staging is determined by the size of the tumor and whether the cancer has spread to the lymph nodes under the arms or to other tissues, such as the lungs, bones, or liver. But you won't know what stage the cancer is in until you have surgery to remove the initial malignant tumor. It is during the surgery, or at a second surgery, that lymph nodes are taken out and biopsied. A node negative result means that your breast cancer is confined to the breast and has not spread to the lymph nodes.

Stage 0

This means carcinoma in situ. The breast tumor is in very early stages and may have been discovered incidentally on a routine mammogram. In this stage, the tumor is confined to the ductal system and has not spread out at all. This stage carries a ten-year survival rate of 98 to 99 percent (meaning that 98 to 99 percent of all women with stage 0 breast cancer live completely cancer-free for at least ten years).

Figure 3.1
FOUR STAGES OF BREAST CANCER

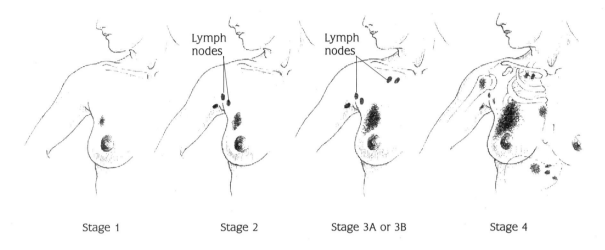

Stage 1   Stage 2   Stage 3A or 3B   Stage 4

Stage 1

This is similar to stage 0, but here, the tumor is invasive and is roughly 2 cm in size, although it is still confined to the breast. Five-year survival rates for stage 1 are now at about 85 to 90 percent.

Stage 2

This could mean a few things: a small tumor (2 cm or less) has spread to the lymph nodes (i.e., you are node positive) but has not metastasized; a larger tumor (2 to 5 cm), which may or may not have spread to the lymph nodes, but has not metastasized; or a large tumor (over 5 cm) hasn't yet spread to the lymph nodes. Stage 2 carries a five-year survival rate of 66 percent.

Stage 3A

This means that you have a large tumor (over 5 cm) that has spread to the lymph nodes or to the chest wall but has not metastasized—and is operable. At this stage, five-year survival rates register at about 50 percent.

Figure 3.2

LYMPH NODES THAT MATTER IN BREAST CANCER

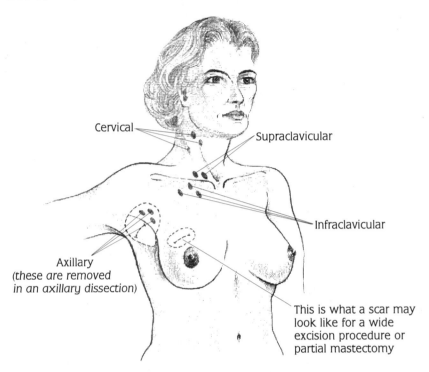

Cervical

Supraclavicular

Infraclavicular

Axillary
*(these are removed
in an axillary dissection)*

This is what a scar may
look like for a wide
excision procedure or
partial mastectomy

Stage 3B

This is a much more serious stage. It means that there is more extensive lymph node involvement, but still no metastasis. However, the tumor may still respond to radiation, chemotherapy, and other non-surgical therapies. Five-year survival rates dip down to about 35 percent.

Stage 4

This means that your tumor has invaded other tissues. You might find a lump around your collar bone, for example, or find that the cancer has spread to your bones, liver, or lungs. Five-year survival rates for stage 4 breast cancer hover around 10 percent. But 80 to 90 percent of breast cancers today are found in either stage 0, stage 1, or stage 2, which means that they respond well to treatment.

A recent study out of Indiana University School of Medicine suggests that if your cancer has spread to other parts of your body, you may have a poorer prognosis if your cancer cells contain a molecule called Her-2, which is made by a specific gene in some breast cancer cells.

Lymph nodes

In addition to the stage classification, successful treatment of both stage 2 and stage 3 (A or B) breast cancer is extremely dependent on the number of positive lymph nodes (i.e., cancerous lymph nodes). See figure 3.2. If you have only one positive lymph node, you're in better shape than if you had four, which is still better than having fifteen positive lymph nodes.

A final, and very crucial, note for all women with stage 3B and stage 4 breast cancer: these survival statistics were compiled prior to the widespread use of chemotherapy, which started being used only twelve years ago. Survivors of breast cancer need to be tracked for at least ten years before new statistics that reflect the success of chemotherapy can be published. In other words, there are no statistical odds against you, because there are no meaningful statistics available yet. In addition, statistics apply to large populations of women, not to individuals. Breast cancer is very heterogeneous: it behaves differently in each individual.

TNM

No, this is not a new cable channel, but a stage classification system currently used by pathologists. TNM stands for tumor, node, metastasis and uses a logical numbering system after each letter to describe the state of affairs in your body. For example, T-1, N-0, M-0 means a small tumor of 0 to 2 cm has been found but you are node negative and free of metastasis. Therefore, your cancer is in stage 1. A report of T-3, N-3, M-0 would put you in stage 3 because the tumor is larger, with positive nodes near the collarbone. Table 3.1 shows an actual TNM chart. If you know the correct size of your tumor (which must be physically measured by a pathologist) and whether you're node-negative or node-positive (this information can be determined only after the pathology report, however), you can calculate your tumor and node class (your T and N class) using the chart.

Table 3.1

TNM STAGING SYSTEM

	Tumor size	Cancer in lymph nodes	Metastases in distant parts of the body
Stage 0	In situ cancer–very localized	No	No
Stage 1	Tumor no larger than 3/4" (2 cm) across	No	No
Stage 2	Tumor is more than 1" across but has not reached chest wall or skin	Tumor may have spread to reach axillary (underarm) lymph nodes	No
Stage 3A	Tumor can be any size but has not reached the chest wall or skin	Tumor has spread to the axillary (underarm) lymph nodes and may have caused these to grow and attach to each other and to nearby tissues	No
Stage 3B	Tumor can be any size but has not reached the chest wall or skin	Tumor may have reached lymph nodes near the breastbone as well as the underarm	No
Stage 4	Tumor can be any size	Tumor has probably spread to lymph nodes	Yes

Source: Brenner, David J., and Eric J. Hall. Making the Radiation Therapy Decision. *Los Angeles: Lowell House, 1996.*

The TNM staging system requires an accurate tumor size to be shown in your pathology report. This is key, which is why an experienced breast surgeon should be the one removing the tumor. A specialist will understand the art of breast surgery and the importance of removing the tumor in one piece as opposed to piecemeal—which has been known to happen. Unless the tumor is removed in one piece, it is difficult to accurately determine its size, and size determines staging. It is important that the pathologist accurately measure the tumor (something that isn't always done, particularly in tumors smaller than 1 cm).

DEALING WITH DIAGNOSIS . . . AND DOCTORS

When you are first told that you have a malignant lump, or that you have cancer, you will experience shock. Shock can be manifested in a variety of reactions, ranging from no reaction at all, or numbness, to high panic, in which your life flashes before your eyes and you can't think straight because your mind is racing in a hundred directions. Psycho-oncolgists—experts in the field of psycho-oncology, who specialize in dealing with patients' emotions and the many psychological issues of cancer diagnosis—classify the initial reaction of diagnosis as immobilization shock or high panic. Another phrase they use is emotion versus no emotion. Denial is also a common reaction (it can't be true, there's been a mistake), but it often centers on denying the seriousness or the urgency of the diagnosis, rather than the diagnosis itself.

Many top breast cancer specialists and cancer survivors stress that a breast cancer diagnosis is *not* an emergency. You do not have to make the decisions regarding your treatment in the next twenty-four hours, or even the next week. It has taken a long time for your cancer to have reached the stage of discovery (somewhere between eight and ten years). As one specialist puts it, diagnosis does not mean that your breast cancer has suddenly developed, it simply means that you know something more about your body than you did a day ago. You should also note that just because a biopsy comes back showing a malignant tumor, it doesn't always mean that the tumor is truly dangerous, as is the case with many in situ tumors.

I promise, two weeks will not make any difference to your overall prognosis or survival. Take the time to absorb the information, to educate yourself about your particular type of cancer (by reading a book like this one), and to get a second opinion. In fact, many cancer centers today have a built-in second opinion structure, where each member of a multidisciplinary team of specialists independently reviews each new diagnosis; the specialists then discuss their findings to make sure they all agree about the diagnosis, staging, and treatment recommendations.

ARE YOU SURE?

If you're experiencing denial, which is a perfectly normal reaction to a breast cancer diagnosis, use the denial to learn more. Here's what you can ask your specialist or any consulting specialist (that is, the second-opinion doctor) to make sure there's no mistake; this will help you deal with the information better. I've taken the liberty of wording the questions in a way that you can use this list as a script in case you're struggling for your own words.

1. I've read that some tumors can look malignant but act benign, and vice versa. Are you sure that my tumor doesn't fall into this category? (Note: The current classification system is definitely flawed, in that it can predict the behavior of tumors on the basis of certain biomarkers, but it can't tell doctors everything there is to know about the biological makeup of each tumor. It's like being able to predict how a baby will react to a loud noise, but knowing you have no way of absolutely knowing how it will in fact react until it actually does.)

2. Are you basing this diagnosis on a single pathology report, or have other specialists reviewed it? (Note: Doctors are cautioned never to accept a single pathology report as the last word and to never tell patients they have cancer on the sole basis of written or oral reports.)

3. Have you discussed my current health status and family history with other oncologists thoroughly so you can recommend an appropriate therapy for me?

4. Has the pathologist reviewed enough samples to make an accurate diagnosis?

5. Are you sure that the tissue samples the pathologist reviewed came from me?

6. Have you reviewed the pathology slides and report yourself? (This is key.

Ask for a copy of the pathology report, and request your doctor to go over it with you and explain the report in language you can understand.)

7. How many cassettes (slides) were made from my biopsy? (Anything less than twenty cassettes per biopsy is a suspiciously low number. Twenty to thirty cassettes will ensure that nothing about the specimen was overlooked.)

8. Which "margins" were involved? (In the same way that a piece of paper has left, right, top, and bottom margins, so does a biopsy. Does the surgeon know if the cancer was closest to the nipple [medial], head [superior], side [lateral], feet [inferior], skin [anterior], or chest wall [posterior]?)

9. Was my tumor multicentric or multifocal? (This will tell you whether your tumor was isolated or not. More than one tumor in the same quadrant of your breast means that your tumor is multifocal; tumors in more distant quadrants of your breast mean that the tumor is multicentric.)

10. (If you're more comfortable . . .) Can I request a second look at my tissue samples from another institution?

11. (If your doctor doesn't seem to know the answers to a lot of these questions . . .) I'd like to ask the pathologist some questions. Can you give please give me his or her name?

Your specialist should not be annoyed at your questions. If he is, this is a bad sign, and you should try to go elsewhere. In fact, most cancer specialists are more concerned about the patients who don't ask questions (such patients are called passive patients). Unless you ask questions, your specialist has no way of knowing whether he has given you adequate or appropriate information so that you can participate in treatment decisions.

WHO WILL MANAGE MY CANCER TREATMENT?

Doctors work in teams to manage cancer therapy. Your primary care physician, surgeon (for breast surgery), radiation oncologist (in charge of radiation therapy), and medical oncologist (in charge of chemotherapy) are all involved in your treatment.

If you have a lump in your breast, you may be referred to a breast surgeon to have the lump investigated (see Chapter 4). The surgeon will handle everything from the biopsy phases to the actual diagnosis of breast cancer. If it is your family doctor or gynecologist who makes the final breast cancer diagnosis (from a positive biopsy), then he will immediately refer you to either a breast surgeon (often a general surgeon who may specialize in breast cancer). If you're not referred to a breast surgeon, you must insist on it. A gynecologist should never manage your breast cancer treatment.

The breast surgeon will advise you of your treatment options and will assist you in making the treatment decision you're comfortable with; it is not your surgeon's role to make the treatment decision for you, however. For example, the survival rates for a lumpectomy with radiation and for a mastectomy (that is, a modified radical mastectomy) are equal: at least fifteen years. Therefore, other issues such as convenience, fear of recurrence, comfort, quality of life, and so on will factor into your very individual decision. (Breast surgery is discussed on page 112.)

After your surgery, you should be referred to other specialists: a radiation oncologist, who will look after the radiation phase of your treatment, and, possibly, a medical oncologist, who will look after your chemotherapy and hormone therapy treatments. You may only need to see one of these specialists, however. Your breast surgeon will probably be the project manager, coordinating and consulting with both oncologists regarding your progress. In some cases, a family/primary care physician might be the project manager. The physician will be continuously updated on your progress by the specialists; in fact, the physician might be in charge of finding the specialists for you. You may wish to see this doctor regularly for question-and-answer sessions to help you cope with all your treatments. The family/primary care physician may also be a good source for referrals, second opinions, and psychosocial support, even if she is not the project manager.

A word about HMOs (Health Maintenance Organizations)

If you belong to an HMO and your plan doesn't have a breast surgeon, you should try to push the HMO to let you either see a breast surgeon or go to a breast center. Many general surgeons continue to do out-of-date procedures for breast cancer, while a breast surgeon is up-to-speed with the latest literature and with studies on the value of this procedure over that. For example, many surgeons will still perform an axillary (armpit) dissection for ductal carcinoma in situ, even though current literature suggests that this is absolutely not indicated!

What many insurance companies make you do is contact your primary-care physician, who is supposed to initiate a formal request to refer you to a breast specialist, outside the "network" if your health plan's book doesn't include a breast surgeon. This doesn't always work, however. Sometimes insurance companies will still insist that you go to a general surgeon from their list of approved surgeons, telling you to look for one who does "breasts"—which is inappropriate. If you find problems getting to the right specialist, contact one of the breast cancer advocacy groups listed at the back. Many of these groups have secured free legal help through local lawyers, who will help you get the benefits you need.

WHAT SHOULD YOU ASK?

The first thing you'll need to do after your cancer has been diagnosed is to get some answers directly from your project manager, likely your breast surgeon. The best way to get answers is to schedule a separate appointment with the surgeon and use the entire time for a question-and-answer period. Write down all your questions ahead of time and tape record the answers, so you can review them later either by yourself or with a supportive spouse (who should go with you to this appointment), partner, or friend. Often when we're anxious, we don't hear correctly; we misconstrue facts and block out what we don't want to hear. That's why it is important to tape your doctor's answers.

What should you ask? Obviously, questions will vary from person to person, but here are some general ones to get you started. While your surgeon may not be able to answer all the questions in the following list, she can certainly direct you to someone who can answer what she cannot.

1. Find out where you can go for more information, and ask to be referred to a support group or a therapist or social worker who specializes in working with breast cancer patients.

2. Request the doctor to draw you a diagram of the cancerous organ or part and shade in the areas where the cancer is situated or has spread. Visualizing the cancer makes it easy to understand.

3. Ask about the size of the tumor involved, and whether the size was determined from a mammogram or an actual biopsy. If the size of the tumor is greater than 3 cm, neoadjuvant chemotherapy (preoperative chemotherapy) may be done to shrink the tumor so that you can have breast conservation surgery.

4. Ask if the entire tumor was removed when it was biopsied. If it wasn't, what were the margins of the cancer (see page 113)? Can a re-excision be done to make sure that the entire tumor was removed? (This is done frequently by many breast surgeons.)

5. Ask whether the cancer is differentiated or undifferentiated. Breasts can be invaded by either kind of cancer cell.

6. Ask what stage the cancer is in.

7. Ask if your hospital or treatment center has a multidisciplinary breast cancer team. This means that a number of breast cancer specialists—pathologists, surgeons, radiation and medical oncologists—discuss your case together and recommend treatment options.

8. Find out what treatment is being recommended and why. It's important to note that for early stage invasive cancer (stages 1, 2, and even 3), a lumpectomy with or without axillary dissection is as effective as a modified radical mastectomy. However, neoadjuvant (preoperative) chemotherapy is usually done to shrink tumors in a stage 3A or 3B cancer, after which a modified radical mastectomy is performed. So if your surgeon tells you, for instance, that your survival rate is greater with a modi-

fied radical mastectomy for a stage 2 cancer, alarm bells should go off in your head because this is not a recommendation that is up-to-date with current medical literature. You should also find out how many breast conserving surgeries versus mastectomies your surgeon does.

9. Find out how the treatment will help, what risks or side effects are associated with it (including how all this affects your menstrual cycle), and the survival rate of successful treatment.

10. Find out where and when the treatments will take place and how long they'll last. For example, if you're having radiation therapy, find out if it is being done at an accredited facility.

11. What if you miss one treatment? Can you make it up?

12. What other health problems should you be on the look-out for during treatment?

13. How can you contact your managing doctor between visits?

14. Can you take other medications during treatments? Or, how will the treatments affect other medications you're taking?

15. What about alcohol? Considering what you're going through, you might want a glass of wine or a shot of hard liquor occasionally. Is that okay?

16. If you're not given a very good prognosis, find out if you can participate in new studies or clinical trials that are using new drugs or therapies.

17. Find out what will happen to you if you choose not to undergo treatment. For example, if you have an advanced stage of breast cancer and are told that you will most likely not survive, and if chemotherapy treatment is not considered to be significantly useful, you may choose to fight the cancer with a gentler, more holistic approach, so you can enjoy the time you do have left more fully. Many women do not regret this choice.

SECOND (AND THIRD) OPINIONS

Getting a second opinion means that you see two separate doctors about the same biopsy report to check if the diagnoses match. You also see two separate doctors about treatment recommendations to check if the recommendations match. If your tissue samples were carefully analyzed in the first place, you probably won't hear different diagnoses, but when it comes to treatment recommendations, you very well may.

For example, a fifty-year-old woman diagnosed with a stage 1 ductal carcinoma may be told by one surgeon that a lumpectomy (a surgery that removes the tumor but conserves the breast; discussed further on) followed by external radiation therapy (discussed in Chapter 4) is all that's necessary for now. (This is known as local therapy because only the breast is treated.)

Another surgeon may feel that local therapy is inadequate and may advise doing a mastectomy, followed by radiation, chemotherapy, and hormone therapy.

Why the discrepancy? Well, Surgeon 1 feels that since the cancer is only in stage 1, a more conservative approach is just fine, since it will lessen the woman's trauma and preserve her body—something he feels is an important aspect in recovery. Surgeon 2 doesn't want to take any chances: she feels that since the woman's age places her in a higher risk group, she should go after the cancer more aggressively. And there are other approaches to this scenario. A third surgeon may advise a bilateral mastectomy, which involves removing both breasts, followed by radiation, chemotherapy, and hormone therapy. Her reasoning is that there's a strong likelihood of the breast cancer recurring in the other breast down the road, and she wants to prevent a relapse and further trauma to this patient. Let's get rid of this thing now and get this woman on her feet once and for all is how the third surgeon feels.

And you know what? All these approaches are perfectly valid. That's where you come in. Hearing the different approaches will help you choose the therapy that's right for you.

Guidelines for seeking second opinions

It's usually par for the course to get a second opinion in a breast cancer diagnosis. Here are some general guidelines to follow. If you answer yes to any of the following questions, it means you are absolutely justified in getting another opinion.

1. Is the diagnosis uncertain? If your doctor isn't sure what your biopsy results mean, or what stage the cancer is in, you have every right to go elsewhere.

2. Is the diagnosis life-threatening? In this case, hearing the same news from someone else may help you cope better.

3. Is the treatment controversial, experimental, or risky? Since treatment guidelines for breast cancer change rapidly, what's experimental today may be standard therapy tomorrow. Nevertheless, if you're uncomfortable with the recommended treatment, perhaps another doctor can recommend another approach.

4. Is the treatment not working? This is a question that may come up at a later stage in the game. If you have a more advanced stage of breast cancer, for example, you may need to try another approach if you're not responding to a given therapy.

5. Are risky tests or procedures being recommended? If you don't like the sound of a bone marrow transplant, find out if there's an alternative approach.

6. Do you want another approach? An eighty-year-old woman with heart disease and high blood pressure who is diagnosed with advanced breast cancer may die from heart disease or a stroke before she dies from breast cancer, which tends to grow slowly in the elderly. As a result, her doctor may decide that she's too frail for surgery, chemotherapy, or radiotherapy, and opt to leave her alone. The woman may find this approach unacceptable and may demand that her breast cancer be treated. (Treating breast cancer in the elderly is an area of much research right now.)

7. Are you uneasy with your current doctor? Always listen to that little voice in your head that says, there's something that doesn't feel right, here.

8. Is the doctor competent? A qualified breast surgeon should be doing roughly two to three breast surgeries a week. If you have the slightest doubt about your doctor's ability, go somewhere else—this will either reaffirm your faith in your doctor or confirm your original suspicions.

The alarm bells

The following procedures should make alarm bells go off in your head and get you to another doctor fast.

- *Preventive or prophylactic surgery.* Sometimes, given a family with a long history of breast or ovarian cancer, doctors may suggest removing the breasts and ovaries before any cancer surfaces. Get another opinion if this is suggested.
- *Mastectomy.* Often, a lumpectomy is all that's necessary for an early breast cancer. It is important to get another opinion, however. You may very well need a mastectomy after all, but it's best to check.
- *Radical mastectomy (a.k.a. the Halsted mastectomy).* This procedure, which is mutilating to say the least, is needed only in rare cases. Again, be sure that it's necessary.

HOW TO USE A SPECIALIST

Depending on where you live, you may or may not have the luxury of shopping for a specialist the way you do for a family doctor because you're usually referred to one only when you need one. And in smaller centers (particularly in Canada), there may not be any choice in specialists at all. Your main concern is getting better as soon as possible, and getting to see another specialist in some places can take months—time you really can't afford when you're ill. Here are some guidelines which will help you make maximum use of your specialist:

1. Tape record your visit. Specialists often say a lot in a small space of time. When you're upset or overwhelmed by all the information being hurled at you, you may not hear what the specialist is saying. Tape recording the visit is helpful because you can replay the information when you're more relaxed, and thus better understand what you've been told.
2. Take along a family member or a friend to the appointment. That way, you have support while you're there, and you can also discuss the information with someone who may have heard more of the discussion.
3. Take a list of questions with you, and tape record the answers. If you have a lot of questions, make a list so you don't forget them. The specialist has an obligation to answer all your questions, and if she doesn't have time, there are some options. Give the specialist your list and ask if she can address

them in your next appointment. If thats not possible, agree on a time when the specialist can call you at home and address the questions. As a final resort, ask if there is a resident studying with the specialist with whom you can arrange a question-and-answer session. (Usually, a resident is a "specialist in training" and can address your questions.)

4. Request literature or videos on your illness from the specialist or the number of a support group, a counselor/therapist, or a support organization that you can call for more information.

5. Ask the specialist to draw you a diagram of your illness.

DEALING WITH THE C-WORD

The most difficult part of a cancer diagnosis is dealing with the notion of actually having cancer. Your feelings about the diagnosis will obviously depend on the severity of your cancer and the statistical reality of survival. But even if you're assured repeatedly that your cancer is curable, the stigma of cancer is still there. To make matters worse, cancer patients often find that they spend most of their time reassuring other people that everything will be okay, particularly close family members and relatives. By the time they finish comforting them, and dispelling the third-party panic that results, they have very little energy left for themselves. Pity is another problem. When others are anxious about your condition and worry about how it will affect them, or fear the same predicament, their response is pity—the I-would-hate-for-that-to-be-me attitude. Nobody likes to be pitied, of course. When people are supportive, however, their sympathy implies a do unto others philosophy.

So what can you do to avoid the panic and pity of others? First, get as much information as you can about your condition before you begin to tell people other than close family members about your illness. For information and access to networks of other cancer or patients, you can ask your own doctors or contact breast cancer support groups or foundations in your area. (Review the list at back of this book for suggestions.) Clinics and hospitals have social workers, psychologists, therapists, and support groups who exclusively work with cancer patients. Ask your doctor to refer you to one of these professionals. It's important to talk to someone who has had experience with other cancer patients, as well as to women who are going through, or have gone through, the same kind of cancer as you. That way, your own experience won't feel so isolating, and it can be put in perspective.

Or, you can turn to other support networks. For example, many corporations and businesses now offer a free program to their employees called the Employee Assistance Program. If you have access to this program, you can speak to a qualified therapist in complete confidence and at your own convenience while your employer picks up the tab. These sessions are prepaid, and the program is offered as a benefit and service to employees. If your company provides the Employee Assistance Program, brochures or posters for the program will be displayed on company bulletin boards with a 1-800 number. If you're not sure whether the program is provided, ask the human resources manager. Do take advantage of it if you can. Depending on your religious or community affiliations, you may want to go to a social service organization that your community funds. These organizations have social workers or therapists on hand; and many women find turning to clergy comforting.

Only after you've done some of your own research, gathered some answers, or spoken to someone about your cancer will you be equipped to tell people about your condition.

Who can you tell?

What you say is as important as who you tell. That's why it is better to break the news about your condition when you are calmer and less frightened yourself. If you're married or in a relationship, your partner and children are the most obvious people on your list. I will discuss this at greater length below. But there are usually other people you need to think about in addition to very close family members.

When you're ready to tell, it's important to first tell people who are supportive. Figuring out who is supportive isn't always easy, of course. Patient-support experts recommend using what they call secret rules. If you had an important secret to reveal about yourself, who would you tell? Someone you trust unconditionally. Secondly, it's important to ask yourself what the purpose of telling John or Jane is and what you can expect John or Jane's reaction to be. This may help prepare you for various responses.

I often say that cancer is like a wedding: it can bring out the worst in some people and the best in others. For instance, people who you think are supportive friends can say the most terrible and inappropriate things. The same goes for family members. Meanwhile, the most caring and supportive people can pop out from the most unlikely places; acquaintances from work, public transit buddies, or fifth cousins twice removed who call you after they hear the news through the grapevine. But you will often find the best support in a breast cancer support group, where you can talk with other women who are going through the same thing as you are. Cancer survivors highly recommend this form of communication and support.

Making a list

After you've been diagnosed, make a list of who you must tell and who you should tell. There's a difference. For example, if you have dependent children and/or a spouse, they must be told. Generally, your parents must be told (unless they're estranged or very old and the news would not do them any good). Anyone you live with or have an intimate relationship with must be told. Friends, business associates, and distant relatives, on the other hand, should probably be told, but it's not imperative.

Then, list on a separate sheet of paper who you want to tell. This category usually includes your real friends or one best friend. Sometimes best friends are in fact family members—spouses, mothers, fathers, sisters, adult children (if you're middle aged, for example), aunts, or cousins. Often, best friends are outside the family. When this is the case, they're often more objective and therefore more supportive.

It is this list that becomes your priority: the people you want to tell should be told before the people you must tell. You've chosen them because they're supportive and have proven themselves to you in the past. They will make you feel better, and this will give you strength to tell the people who must know. Bad news is not the same as good news; you don't want to shout it out to the world. This means that the names on your must, should, and want lists differ drastically from the bad news list.

When you're prepared to tackle your want list, make sure you choose your words carefully. For example, instead of saying, "I have cancer," why not begin with, "I have to have an operation." Then lead slowly into the reasons for the operation. That way, the information is presented in a logical sequence, rather than an emotional sequence. The idea is to prevent the person from panicking because it will only make you feel more anxious. You can work on how to present your news by role-playing with your therapist. Or, if you have an open relationship with your doctor, you can discuss how to best present the news with him or her.

After you've told the people on your want list, you could ask them to be with you when you tell the people on your must list. That way, you have support should someone take the news badly.

As for those on the should list, ask someone else to tell them—either someone on your must list or someone on your want list. That way, you don't have the extra burden of speaking to people you're not that close to or don't feel like telling yourself. Sometimes, once you have told the people close to you about your condition, you may wish to simply disregard the should list. Usually, people on the should list are told out of politeness or out of a forced sense of loyalty. Unless there's a very good reason to tell them about your diagnosis, don't. If you have to explain absences to business associates or co-workers, why not just tell them you're going to the doctor for some routine tests. That's all you have to say. Otherwise, rumors and gossip may result. (Unfortunately, other people's misfortunes make the best gossip.)

What if you don't want anyone to know? Depending on your situation, that's okay, too (but it's a good idea to at least speak to a social worker). If you're older, are without a spouse, or have grown children, you may not have to say anything. But most of us don't have the luxury of complete privacy.

Telling a spouse

Breast cancer affects your entire family. It's important to keep in mind that your spouse will be going through as much fear and shock as you. But in some ways, your spouse may be experiencing an even greater feeling of helplessness because there's nothing he can do to make it better or make it go away. But if you hide your own feelings for fear that they will frighten your spouse, a communication breakdown can develop. So try not to do this; try to be honest about your feelings, because this helps to include your spouse in the process. Telling your spouse what he can do for you, around the house or in general, will make him feel as though he's capable, even in a small way, of lessening your burden. It is also important to share what you are going through whenever you need to talk. Indeed, you may find that initially the atmosphere in the home changes hourly and revolves around you. (Are you okay? Do you want to talk now?) Go with the flow and try not to be angry with a continuous checking-in. This is your family's way of caring, and you need to let yourself be cared for. In fact, giving yourself permission is perhaps the hardest thing to do after a breast cancer diagnosis: permission to feel bad; permission to feel needy; permission to let others care for you.

Of course, there are some exceptions to the rule. Some spouses may not have any coping skills to deal with the situation and may even get angry about the diagnosis or leave the house to work it out. Obviously, this is a sign that there are fundamental problems in your relationship anyway; the diagnosis is not causing this behavior, it's simply bringing the truth about the relationship to the surface faster. In these cases, family therapy, counseling, and spousal cancer support groups (support groups for the spouses of cancer patients) can help you resolve your feelings about the diagnosis in a healthy way. Chapter 6 covers spousal support issues in much more detail.

Telling small children

Small children are intuitive beings who will sense that something is wrong in the home. In fact, hiding the diagnosis from a small child is the worst thing you can do because it may lead the child to conclude that she is the cause of your illness. Cancer therapists recommend explaining the situation to children in language they can understand, and, if necessary, explaining or retelling repeatedly. Younger children tend to ask the same questions over and over again. This is their way of finding their bearings in a new situation—hearing the same response helps to build consistency into a new reality.

The well partner or spouse should continue his routine with the children and watch for behavior changes. For example, young children may suddenly have difficulty at school, difficulty sleeping, increased tantrums, separation anxiety from the well or ill parent, or may suddenly start drawing pictures of monsters attacking the ill parent.

No matter how well you explain your illness, or how open you are with your child, exceptions apply, and some children will have more difficulty adjusting. You should seek out family and child counseling if you're worried about a child's behavior.

TREATMENT DECISIONS

Again, a diagnosis of breast cancer is not an emergency. It is important to understand all your treatment options before you make your decision.

Treatment of breast cancer falls into two categories: local, in which only the breast is treated and which involves surgery and often external radiation therapy, and systemic, in which the whole body is treated and which may involve chemotherapy, hormone therapy with the drug tamoxifen, and immuno-complementary therapy to boost the immune system.

Not all breast cancer specialists will recommend the same treatment route for one case. The core difference in treatment philosophies revolves around the issue of adjuvant therapy. Adjuvant therapy involves using systemic treatment after local treatment—even when there is no indication that a cancer has spread. In many ways, adjuvant therapy is considered an insurance policy against future recurrence, and it has been a successful approach for some breast cancer patients, but too high a compromise on quality of life for others. Adjuvant therapy is discussed in detail in Chapter 4.

BREAST SURGERY

You will need some kind of breast surgery no matter what kind of breast cancer you have. The only time surgery isn't offered is when a breast cancer is caught in a very advanced stage. In this case, there is an immediate move toward systemic therapies. But for the majority of women, breast cancer will be discovered anywhere from stage 0 to 2, and surgery will be the first step.

Back in the 1960s and 1970s, no matter how local and early stage a breast cancer was, the only breast cancer surgery that was performed was a crude, disfiguring procedure known as the Halsted radical mastectomy, named after William Halsted, the surgeon who developed the technique in the 1890s. The procedure was for a long time the only known cure for breast cancer, and many women are alive today thanks to it. But about twenty-five years ago, as researchers discovered more about how cancer spreads, more moderate breast surgeries were developed that could be combined with systemic therapies. In addition, due to the efforts of thousands of breast cancer survivors, the negative emotional effects of the Halsted procedure were starting to sink in, giving rise to breast conservation procedures.

Unfortunately, breast conservation procedures may not be your best bet if a recurrence of breast cancer is highly suspected. But many women choose this kind of surgery at first and undergo further surgery if and when a recurrence develops. Other women feel more comfortable with a more radical operation.

For the most part, the old Halsted radical mastectomy has no role in stage 0 to 3 breast cancers. As for modified radical mastectomies, studies show that the overall survival rate of breast cancer patients who underwent the procedure is the same as for those who underwent more conservative surgeries combined with radiation therapy.

If you live in a smaller community, you may not be offered a choice of procedures. In this case, you should definitely get a second opinion before you accept a mastectomy (modified or radical) as the only option. Review the list of questions on page 104 as well.

Breast conservation procedures

The most commonly known surgery that preserves the breast is called a lumpectomy (really a "tumorectomy"). In a lumpectomy, only the breast lump is removed; the rest of the breast tissue and surrounding lymph nodes are left intact. See figure 3.3.

When some normal breast tissue surrounding the lump is removed but the breast and surrounding lymph nodes are left intact, the procedure is referred to by surgeons as a wide excision or a wide lumpectomy (shown in figure 3.3). Other names get tacked on to this basic description once you start zeroing in on the size and shape of the incision. So terms such as *partial mastectomy* (a.k.a. segmental mastectomy) and *quadrantectomy* (when one-quarter of the breast tissue and skin is removed) refer to the same procedure: removing the lump with some normal surrounding breast tissue. The procedure is done so skillfully that the result is as normal looking a breast as possible.

Only about one-third of breast surgeries are lumpectomies (see below); but two-third of breast surgeries could be lumpectomies in light of the size of the tumor and staging. Many studies definitely show that lumpectomy followed by radiation not only preserves a woman's appearance but does so without comprising survival. In Australia, for example, breast-conserving surgery is considered the "best practice" treatment for most women with early breast cancer, and Australia's National Health and Medical Research Council endorses it fully, complete with guidelines on conservation surgery.

Margins of safety

Breast surgeons will tell you that the label given to the wide excision procedure is not what you should worry about. The most important issue when you talk wide excision is margins. Again, as discussed earlier, tumors have margins like a piece of paper. No matter how wide or thin the lumpectomy's total area is, what's crucial is that the tumor's margins are all clear. For example, if a surgeon removes a tumor that's 2 mm in size, a surrounding margin of about 10 mm of normal breast tissue may be removed to ensure that everything abnormal was taken out.

Figure 3.3

THREE TYPES OF WIDE LUMPECTOMY
(WIDE EXCISION PARTIAL MASTECTOMY PROCEDURES)

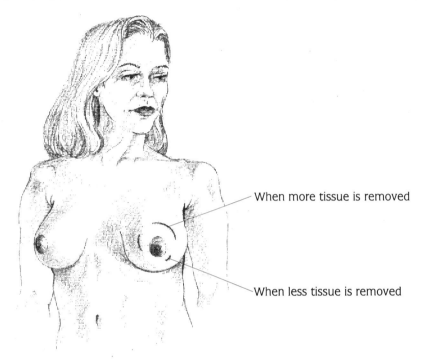

When more tissue is removed

When less tissue is removed

How wide or narrow these margins should be is an issue that is currently being debated by the medical community. One surgeon may argue that a margin of 10 mm for a 2 mm tumor is necessary, while another surgeon may argue that only a 1 mm margin for the same size tumor is sufficient. And then there is the question of how wide a margin should be left for other types of cancers, and whether the margins were classified correctly by the pathologist. The bottom line is this: When you discuss any type of lumpectomy procedure with your doctor, find out exactly what the label being used for the procedure means (such as partial mastectomy, segmental mastectomy, etc.) and have your doctor show you the margins involved by drawing the procedure on paper or using some sort of mannequin to explain what's being done.

Axillary dissection

Axillary dissection sounds terrible, but it merely refers to a procedure in which lymph nodes in the underarm area are removed to make sure they are cancer-free. The word *axilla* literally means armpit. Very often, a partial mastectomy will be combined with an armpit dissection, done separately. The dissection is always done under a general anesthetic because it involves removing anywhere from five to ten nodes. See figure 3.2.

Doctors at the University of South Florida are now using dye and radioactive tracers to help pinpoint which lymph nodes cancer cells are likely to invade, which may mean that axillary lymph node dissection could eventually be eliminated.

Breast removal procedures

Again, depending on the type, location, and stage of your cancer, more radical surgery may be necessary. The least common breast removal surgery is the Halsted radical mastectomy. Most women who need to have a breast removed have a few procedures to choose from, including:

- *Simple mastectomy.* The entire breast is removed, but all muscle tissue and axillary lymph nodes are left alone. This procedure is done when there is a large in situ tumor, but no spread is suspected. Whenever a woman decides to have a preventive mastectomy (to prevent recurrence in the second breast or when familial breast cancer puts a woman at very high risk), a simple mastectomy is done.
- *Subcutaneous mastectomy.* This procedure is not done very often, but it was considered a good idea at one time. Here, the breast skin is preserved, while the breast tissue is dug out through a small incision—akin to pulling a pillow out of a pillow case. Unfortunately, this procedure often doesn't turn out well. First, since about 15 percent of breast tissue is left no matter how carefully the tissue is removed, the purpose of the mastectomy is defeated. Second, reconstructive surgery actually turns out better when you remove the whole breast and start over.

Figure 3.4
MODIFIED RADICAL MASTECTOMY (INSIDE VIEW)

Figure 3.5
MODIFIED RADICAL MASTECTOMY (OUTSIDE VIEW)

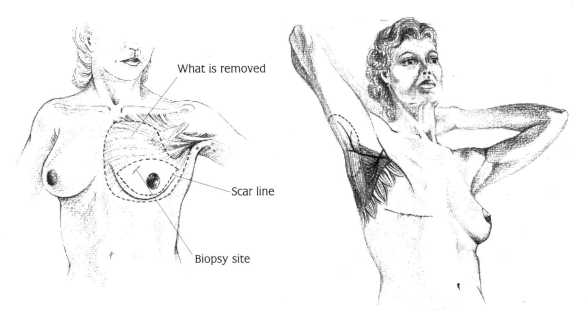

What is removed

Scar line

Biopsy site

- *Modified radical mastectomy (shown in figures 3.4 and 3.5).* Here, the entire breast is removed, along with the axillary nodes, some skin, and the nipple. This procedure is better than the Halsted because it removes fewer surrounding muscles and lymph nodes and also preserves the chest wall muscles and nerves so that the patient is more comfortable afterward.

- *Radical mastectomy (a.k.a. Halsted mastectomy).* This procedure is rarely necessary and is reserved for very advanced breast cancer. It's the same procedure as modified radical mastectomy except that here the pectoralis major and minor chest wall muscles, some nerves, and lymph nodes all the way up to the collarbone are removed. In addition, since so much tissue is removed, a skin graft from another part of the body is taken so that the main chest area can be covered. Again, very few women will ever need this procedure today; in the past, though, every woman with breast cancer had a radical mastectomy.

If you're having a breast removed, you can also have breast reconstructive surgery done at the same time. Chapter 5 discusses breast implants and reconstruction in detail.

QUESTIONS TO ASK BEFORE SURGERY

1. If you're taking any prescription drug whatsoever, make sure you disclose the name of the drug and find out how long before the surgery you need to be off the drug. A class of drugs known as non-steroidal anti-inflammatories (NSAIDs) can be particularly dangerous.

2. The same rules that apply to prescription drugs apply to any over-the-counter drug, be it ibuprofen, acetaminophen, or aspirin.

3. Ask about the likelihood of needing a blood transfusion. If there is a good chance of it, you may wish to consider what's called autologous transfusion, when you give your own blood prior to surgery so that it can be used during your procedure should you require blood. This could reduce the possibility of infection as well as the demand on the public blood supply. There is now a drug called recombinant human erythropoietin that is used to reduce the need for a blood transfusion. This drug is identical to the body's erthropoetin (the hormone that manufactures red blood cells) and increases the red cell count before surgery. Your surgeon will fill you in on the details.

4. Find out how long you need to fast (if you need to, that is) prior to your surgery, what foods you should stay away from before and after the procedure, and so on. Usually you will be told to have your last solids six hours prior to surgery and your last liquids three hours prior to surgery.

WHAT TO EXPECT IN MAJOR SURGERY

Not every woman will need major surgery for a lumpectomy or wide excision, but even for an axillary dissection a general anesthetic and same-day discharge is the norm. Nevertheless, most women will not want to witness the surgery and may prefer a general anesthesia for even a simple lumpectomy. Discuss your anesthesia options with your surgeon prior to the procedure.

As soon as the cancer is detected, your surgery date will be booked—if you've opted for surgery. Most breast surgery is done on a same-day basis. That means that you will be admitted to the hospital a few hours before your surgical procedure, but all your preoperative lab work (blood tests, etc.) will be done on an out-patient basis (you go the hospital or breast center for your tests and then go home). A thorough medical history will be taken by your private physician (a specialist or your family doctor) in his or her office about a week before your surgery.

You will also need to sign a form prior to surgery. This form is a legal document, and make sure you read it before you sign it. If you're having a lumpectomy and the form says partial mastectomy, make sure you ask for a clarification before you sign it. Don't sign the form until all your questions are answered. (Forms vary from state to state, province to province, country to country.)

If you're going under a general anesthetic, you will meet with an anesthesiologist either before your surgery or on the day of your surgery. The anesthesiologist will ask questions to clarify certain information and will also walk you through the surgical procedure, outlining any risks associated with the anesthetic and telling you what to expect when you go under and when you wake up.

If you're having a general anesthetic, once you check into the hospital, you'll be given an intravenous injection to induce sleep before the actual anesthetic is given. You will be awakened for your procedure and wheeled into the operating room. By this point, you will be very groggy and will see everything in a dream-like, half-conscious state.

The area to be operated will be painted with antiseptic. The anesthesiologist will then start the anesthetic via intravenous injection.

When you wake up, you'll be in the recovery room after having been in surgery between one and eight hours (one hour for a lumpectomy; two hours for a mastectomy; six to eight hours for a mastectomy and reconstruction). Some people feel nauseated after an anesthetic and throw up for the first few hours after they wake up. This is normal. The area that was operated will have a dressing. You may not have any feeling in the dressed area because nerve endings are severed during surgical procedures. (They take several years to grow back.) You'll also find a suction tube inserted close to the area that was operated. This tube is connected to either a suction machine (not widely used anymore) or a portable plastic device that is either pinned to your hospital gown or hangs neatly around your neck. The tube drains the area and sucks out all the fluid that collects after surgery. Most hospitals will send you home when you are more alert with bathing instructions to keep the bandaged area dry.

If you have had lymph nodes removed from your underarm, your shoulder may be sore, and you may need to visit a physiotherapist who will help you regain your strength and movement. Many women are discharged before the results of the pathology are in; pathology reports can take anywhere from one to five days to be completed. In this case, you'll see your surgeon at a separate appointment after your surgery when you will go over the pathology report in detail (how invasive the cancer was/is, whether they got it all, the results of your lymph node biopsies and so on). The surgeon will also discuss the next stop on the treatment train with you. The best recovery rules for both lumpectomies and mastectomies are rest, relaxation, and re-evaluation. Your body and your soul need to recover from cancer surgery.

· · · · · · ·

There is life after surgery, but it's a different life from the one you had before the surgery. This life may include radiation therapy, adjuvant therapy such as chemotherapy or hormone therapy, as well as complementary medicine (which you may want to practice for the rest of your life). And your life may include different friends, a different diet, or a different approach to living. The point is that there are many different kinds of lives available after surgery, but you need to choose what works for you. These issues are addressed in the next chapter.

CHAPTER 4

LIFE AFTER SURGERY

This chapter not only discusses the symptoms you will encounter after breast surgery, but the various treatments that follow breast surgery. This includes adjuvant radiation therapy (still considered part of the local treatment), as well as adjuvant systemic therapy, which may involve chemotherapy and hormone therapy. Diet, follow-up appointments, and insurance issues are also discussed.

Many of you may also choose complementary medicine and its holistic approach to cancer. Complementary medicine can be found through non-Western-trained healers and medical practitioners. In cancer therapy, the word *complementary* has come to replace *alternative* because many oncologists are seeing a clear benefit of combining Western and non-Western therapies, that is, you don't have to substitute one kind of healing for another. The more healing that goes on, the better! Complementary medicine is discussed in detail in Chapter 7; it is a route that many women with breast cancer are eagerly seeking out. Reconstructive surgery, which can be done at the same time as breast cancer surgery, is discussed in detail in Chapter 5.

As for your sex life and future fertility, you'll find a discussion of surgical menopause (i.e., menopause that results from medical treatment) within this chapter. The lifestyle issues concerning sexuality and fertility are covered in detail in Chapter 6—along with the special issues that concern the sexual partners of breast cancer patients.

HOW DO YOU FEEL?

When you go under a general anesthetic, a breathing tube is inserted down your throat during surgery. This can cause you to have a sore throat after surgery. If you've had a more extensive breast surgery that involved axillary dissection or the removal of a breast, you'll have drains inserted into the areas that were operated on to remove fluids. (These fluids are postsurgical "gunk" that build up after any operation.) Any pain you're feeling from your procedure, however, can be treated with painkillers.

As for your stitches (a.k.a. sutures), it is common these days to use dissolvable stitches—that is, stitches that are reabsorbed into your skin. For more extensive procedures, it is common to use non-absorbable staples (which don't leave stitch marks) or regular stitches (usually in areas you can't see), both of which will be removed anywhere from seven to ten days after your surgery.

SCARRING

Because most breast surgeries use plastic surgery techniques to "close," scarring isn't as big a problem as the overall appearance of the breast. A modified radical mastectomy will leave you without a breast on one side, a more disturbing sign than any redness from a scar. Partial mastectomy will leave the breast looking as intact and normal as possible, often without any visible signs of surgery other than some redness around the scar. The redness takes about a year to disappear; you have to wait for new skin to grow over it.

If you're alarmed by the appearance of your breast after surgery, you can opt for the several reconstructive procedures that are now available (implant and non-implant), discussed in detail in Chapter 5.

PAIN

Depending on what type of surgery you've had, you may experience a bruise type of pain around your incision or scarline. Painkillers can take care of this, but after a few weeks, you may actually feel a tightness around the area.

You may also suffer from numbness in the area that was operated (your armpit or the chest wall) if any nerve endings were severed during surgery. For the most part, this is a permanent numbness because nerve endings take several years to grow back. Sometimes numb areas may have some tingling from rekindled nerve endings, but the overall feeling you had prior to surgery is rarely restored. More severe side effects include a loss of movement in the shoulder area on the surgery side. This is when physiotherapy comes into play: it helps strengthen your surgery side so you can resume normal movement.

UNDERARM RESISTANCE

There may be some special complications in store for you if you've had an axillary dissection (lymph nodes removed from the armpits). Normally, the lymph nodes under your arms act as drains for all tissue fluid from the arm. Once it is drained through the lymph nodes, this fluid flows back into circulation. This is how you recover from cuts, insect bites, or infections on your hand, fingers, or arm. But when these lymph nodes are removed, or sometimes just blocked by scar tissue, tissue fluid may collect, causing your underarm and arm to swell. This condition is referred to by a number of names: edema (meaning to swell), lymphedema (lymph swelling), or arm edema (swollen arm). No matter what name is used to describe the condition, it is painful and sometimes a little disfiguring when it has flared up. Edema can occur immediately after surgery and then resolve itself, or it may occur fifteen to twenty years after surgery.

The more extensive your surgery was under the arms, the more vulnerable you are to this problem. In fact, surgeons report that when breast conserving procedures are used (see Chapter 3), lymphedema isn't as common as it is with a mastectomy. Furthermore, if you are having radiation on your armpit area, arm edema can really be exacerbated. (Radiation therapy is discussed in detail on page 132.)

Preventing arm edema (lymphedema)

Lymphedema may a be short-lived condition following surgery (known as acute lymphedema) or it may be a chronic condition (chronic lymphedema). The risks of both acute and chronic lymphedema can be reduced if certain

Figure 4.1
ARM EDEMA OR LYMPHEDEMA

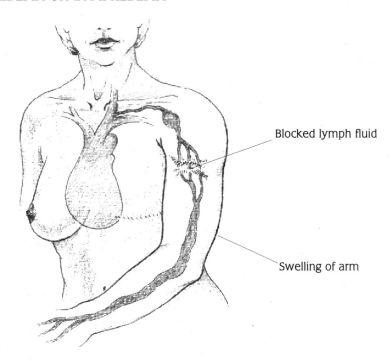

Blocked lymph fluid

Swelling of arm

activities are avoided. Here is a set of guidelines that some experts recommend you follow for the rest of your life. Others say it depends on how extensive your surgery was; you may only need to follow these guidelines for the first couple of weeks immediately after your surgery or while undergoing radiation.

1. *Avoid punctures, cuts, burns, and insect bites on the surgery side.* Any of these things can cause your arm to swell or a serious infection to develop due to improper draining of fluid. Simple precautions like wearing oven mitts every time you go near a hot stove or putting on gardening gloves when you are working outside can eliminate many of the scrapes and cuts you thought nothing of in the past. If you bite your nails or pick the skin around your nails on the surgery side, stop! Also, wear long sleeves whenever you go outside for long periods in warm weather so that you can protect yourself from sunburn and insect bites. Lifelong caution is suggested here.

2. *Avoid having blood taken from your treated side, and avoid having blood pressure cuffs on the treated side.* Lifelong caution is suggested.

3. *Use pectoral muscles with caution.* Any activity or exercise that uses pectoral muscles (be it the breast stroke or ironing) should not exceed fifteen minutes. Use a timer if you can't keep track, and do something entirely different afterwards.

4. *Avoid scrubbing movements.* Whether you're sanding furniture, cleaning a broiler pan with a scouring pad, or scrubbing out the tub—wait at least six weeks after your surgery before you resume these activities because they put a real strain on your upper body.

5. *Take frequent breaks from keyboarding.* If you can master being a one-hand inputter, even better. Otherwise, spending long hours keyboarding may aggravate matters. And remember to "mouse" with the non-surgery hand to reduce shoulder strain.

6. *Take breaks from repetitive arm movements.* Whether you work in a Chrysler plant, are snow-shoveling your driveway, or raking leaves, don't do anything repetitive with your surgery-side arm for more than fifteen minutes without taking a break.

7. *Raise your hand once in a while.* If you know how to raise your hand to answer a question, you can prevent arm edema. Basically, you need to raise your arm enough so that your wrist and elbow are higher than your shoulder. This will help the fluid drain downward. Do this anywhere you are—at home, at the office, or when travelling (try to get a window seat on the surgery side to help elevation). These precautions may need to be employed lifelong.

If you're experiencing swelling...

1. *Lift with the opposite arm.* If you have small children who require lots of carrying around, try to keep your surgery side free from lifting and carrying by imagining that you're on the telephone with that hand.

2. *Carry anything with a strap on the opposite shoulder.* This includes handbags, portable computers, and luggage. If you need both shoulders to carry it, consider getting a pushcart, airport style.

3. *Carry anything with a handle with the opposite hand.* This includes brief-cases and shopping bags. Again, pushcarts might be necessary if you have a lot of stuff to schlep.

4. *Push, don't pull.* Pushing items with the surgery-side hand is fine, but pulling is not. This includes golf carts, vacuum cleaners, baby carriages, shopping carts, and luggage with wheels. If you must pull, use the opposite side of your body.

5. *No push-ups.* This exercise puts tremendous strain on your shoulders and chest muscles. It is wise to wait three to six months after surgery before you resume this exercise. No "unintentional" push-ups, either.

WHEN DO YOU NEED PHYSIOTHERAPY?

If you've had surgery or radiation under your arms, or have had more extensive breast surgery (such as a modified radical mastectomy), you will benefit from physiotherapy, which can reduce arm edema, or help you regain regular movement on your surgery side. If you are feeling perfectly fine and have regular movement on both sides, you may want to simply consult with a physiotherapist after your surgery just to go over okay versus not-okay activities.

A common problem with more extensive surgery is poor shoulder movement on the surgery side. Some women develop what's known as tethering, where the tissues under the skin connect in ways God never intended. It feels like tight ropes under your arm, even your wrists can feel restricted. Tethering can be eased with physiotherapy and a variety of slow stretches.

FATIGUE

A typical day in the life of a woman recovering from breast cancer surgery involves a collapse on the couch after a brief outing or errand. And this comes as quite a shock. In fact, many breast cancer patients list fatigue as one of the most frustrating postoperative symptoms. That's why, even though you may feel fine at seven in the morning and feel like putting in a full day's work, you may want to give yourself some time to rest.

A common scenario is to plan a day's worth of activities and find that you can only accomplish one or two before total exhaustion sets in. This fatigue is not caused so much by the surgery as it is by the events surrounding surgery: stress, re-organization of lifestyle, decisions about postsurgical treatment (adjuvant therapy), waiting for biopsy results, and dealing with concerned friends and family. Your body is also responding to recent changes in *its* environment, be it the removal of axillary lymph nodes or the removal of tissue.

The remedy for fatigue is obvious: rest! But finding the time to rest can be challenging. Here are some tips:

1. Forget "banking hours"—keep "toddler hours." Get up early and have a nice breakfast. (This is the best time to get things done!) Nap mid-morning. Nap after lunch. Have an early dinner, followed by "bathtime," and go to bed by eight after reading a good story.

2. If you need to work for a living like most women on the planet, try to arrange flex time so you can work early and get home early. You will have much more energy in the early morning and get pooped out by early afternoon. You'll also avoid rush hour, which can tire anybody out. Or else, try to build in time for a nap and go back to the office later.

3. Limit your errands. Shop and bank by phone; use couriers to save yourself running back and forth; divide up errands between family members and friends.

4. Limit visitors and visiting. Visit places and people that give you energy. In other words, say yes to that "chick flick" with a good friend; no to that dysfunctional family brunch you promised your aunt you'd attend.

5. Next time someone asks, "Is there anything I can do," ask the kind soul to run an errand you don't have the energy for!

6. Make a list of everything that needs to get done. Then cut it in half until only what must get done that day gets done. Anything that can wait, should.

ADJUVANT THERAPY

The word *adjuvant* comes from the Latin word *aiding*. In the context of breast cancer, adjuvant therapy is defined in a number of ways by oncologists. Many simply refer to any treatment following surgery as adjuvant therapy, meaning additional therapy. Other oncologists refer to preventive or prophylactic therapy as adjuvant therapy: your life doesn't depend on it right now, but the therapy is there just in case. Some oncologists refer to adjuvant therapy as treatment that prevents recurrence; you may as well go in for it now before the cancer revives itself and attacks again. And still others simply use adjuvant therapy as insurance: the more you buy now, the greater your protection. But no matter how your oncologist defines adjuvant therapy, it boils down to one or all of the following:

- *Radiotherapy.* Discussed in detail on pages 131–136, radiotherapy is the use of external radiation beams to genetically alter any cancer cells left in the body. (Occasionally, radiotherapy is recommended before surgery.)
- *Chemotherapy.* Discussed on pages 136–151, chemotherapy will be recommended any time the cancer is suspected of being invasive. As discussed in Chapter 3, if your cancer was discovered in stage 3, you may be advised to have chemotherapy prior to surgery.
- *Hormone therapy.* Discussed on pages 150–152, hormone therapy is used when the cancer is more invasive, in that you have positive lymph nodes and the cancer cells are estrogen-receptor positive, meaning that they seem to thrive on estrogen. You may be offered an estrogen-blocking drug such as tamoxifen, or other therapies.
- *The combo platter.* All three therapies may be recommended, depending on the stage and type of breast cancer.

WHAT'S THE BENEFIT PACKAGE?

This is the first question you need to ask your practitioners before you say yes to any of these therapies. Often, there are no tangible benefits to the therapies so you can look back a year later and say, "Gee, I'm so glad I did that!" That's where playing the numbers game really comes in handy.

For example, after your surgery for an in situ cancer, you have a very good chance of living cancer-free for the rest of your life; chemotherapy may not raise the odds significantly at all. In this case, you'd be trading in about six months of health and normal life for chemotherapy's side effects without getting a return on your investment. Is this a benefit? Many women would say no. On the other hand, if you're not going to have peace of mind unless you have the chemotherapy, you might decide that, for you, the therapy is beneficial so that you can feel that you did everything you could to ensure your survival.

Jane Doe versus Joan Doe

Adjuvant therapy is an incredibly personal decision that has as much to do with your psychological makeup and personal value system as the physical cancer. What Jane Doe considers a benefit may be Joan Doe's idea of a nightmare. So you need to be clear in your mind about what quality of life means to you. For Jane, quality of life may mean peace of mind; for Joan Doe, it may mean living life without invasive treatment. Furthermore, even though Jane and Joan both have a 75 percent chance of living cancer-free for the rest of their lives (twenty to thirty years, say), Jane may want to up the odds to 95 percent with chemotherapy, while Joan may feel that 75 percent are great odds and may walk away feeling satisfied with partial surgery and radiation.

Weighing the benefits

You should never feel forced into having—or not having—adjuvant therapy unless you are comfortable with your choice. By asking the following questions of yourself and your doctors, you should be able to arrive at a decision you can live with.

1. *How will treatment affect my day-to-day life?* Questions about fatigue, traveling to the treatment center, sex life, childcare, and so on, are all valid. Find out!
2. *Will this treatment prolong my life (if so, by how much) or permanently eradicate the cancer?* In the final analysis, are you gaining years of life or reassurance? Know the true statistical benefits.

3. *How does my age affect the outcome of this treatment?* For example, chemotherapy seems to be of greater benefit to premenopausal women than postmenopausal women, while hormone therapy is of greater benefit to postmenopausal women than premenopausal women. The interplay between the ovaries and these treatments seems to be the crux of the matter, but no one can really explain why. So far, theories and studies are conflicting.

4. *What are the short-term side effects of this treatment?* Nausea, vomiting, and hair loss are examples of "short-term" side effects.

5. *What are the long-term side effects of this treatment?* Premature ovarian failure, followed by menopause and permanent sterility, is an example of a "long-term" side effect of chemotherapy (if you're premenopausal); a risk of liver and endometrial cancer is a "long-term" side-effect of tamoxifen. Get all this information up front before you sign on the dotted line.

6. *Is this treatment covered by my insurer?* If so, how will this treatment affect future coverage and my overall policy? If you lose your insurance coverage over not-very-tangible benefits, you may want to reconsider. (This is not a concern if you live in Canada—as of 1997.)

7. *How will this treatment affect my immune system?* This is a crucial question. Chemotherapy, in particular, will suppress your immune system, leaving you vulnerable to infections and viruses you may never have had before.

8. *How will this treatment affect my job or future employment?* In essence, how much time will you need to take off work, and how much time can you afford to take off? Do you have long-term disability benefits? Can you take a leave of absence? And so on.

9. *Can some "timelines" for the entire adjuvant treatment process be mapped out?* Take a daytimer or wall calendar into your doctor's office and literally plan the timing of the various therapies. Seeing it down on a calendar will help you decide whether or not it is feasible.

10. *What dietary changes should I be making to complement these treatments?* It's amazing how many people forget to ask this question, and

how many doctors forget to tell patients about diet during various treatments. See Chapter 10 for more information on nutritional guidelines and Chapter 7 for more information on complementary medicine.

RADIATION THERAPY

Radiation therapy involves the use of high-energy X rays or gamma rays (also referred to as cobalt radiation). X rays and gamma rays use photons (a photon has a different "dosage" of energy than light) to penetrate the skin. Radiation therapy is not chemotherapy—your hair will not fall out unless your scalp is being radiated. Radiation treatment is very exact and directs radiation only at areas where the cancer has spread.

The concept of radiation is very simple. Radiation alters the DNA of the cancer cell's nucleus (center). The actual process is a little more complex. First, you'll be referred to a radiation oncologist, an oncologist who specializes in radiation therapy. (This is not to be confused with a radiologist—a doctor who specializes in reading X rays and diagnostic test results.)

Radiation therapy is given over a long period of time rather than all at once, because the dose involves a fine balance: enough radiation to destroy cancer cells but not to destroy your healthy tissue, which, in a sense, is in the way of the beam. Certain cancer cells are more sensitive to radiation than others, in the same way that some cockroaches respond to poison while others don't.

When radiation therapy is given as adjuvant therapy to help prevent the cancer from recurring, the treatment scenario is usually as follows: one to three minutes of radiation every weekday for three-and-half weeks to six weeks. Most patients have external radiation (meaning a beam aimed at the outside flesh). However, there are special cases where internal radioactive implants are surgically placed directly inside a tumor; this is discussed more on page 137.

Reasons to radiate

Radiation therapy is not just adjuvant therapy, but local therapy. In other words, it doesn't involve your whole body—just the part that is cancerous. Any time you have a breast-conserving procedure, such as the various types of partial mastectomies discussed in Chapter 3, external adjuvant radiation therapy will be offered to you as the second half of your local therapy.

Radiation therapy will also be the next step after more advanced cancer surgery, particularly if the doctors suspect that the cancer has spread.

Radiation therapy is occasionally the first stop in treatment when breast cancer is in a very advanced stage (beyond stage 3A, usually). In this case, radiation is used to help shrink the tumor so surgery can be performed.

Finally, radiation therapy is used as a palliative measure in more advanced stages of breast cancer, not so much to cure the cancer, but to simply help relieve symptoms when a cancer has metastasized into other areas such as lymph nodes and bones.

The dress rehearsal

Before you actually have your radiation treatments, you'll need to have a "simulation" exercise run, so that the equipment, dosage, and target area can be precisely determined. So you'll undergo a mock session with a "simulator" machine that looks like the actual radiation machine used in treatment, but isn't. Data is collected about your size, body shape, and the location and extent of the area that needs to be treated. The simulator also determines what kind of shieldings you'll need for the parts of your body not receiving radiation.

Getting tattooed

As shown in figure 4.2, the radiation oncologist will either mark you with a "permanent" marker that wears off after a few weeks, or tattoo you by injecting tiny dots of special dye in precise areas he has already marked off in washable ink during the simulation. This dye will later be picked up by the radiation beam, which will use the tattoo as an exact target for a squared-off section, predetermined by the radiation oncologist. The tattoo is permanent, but fortunately is not very noticeable: the dots are the size of a freckle.

A few days after you are tattooed, you will report to a radiation clinic. Radiation clinics are usually located in the hospital basement because hospitals want to minimize the risk of healthy people being exposed to radiation. But reporting to a clinic in the bowels of a hospital may feel isolating and depressing.

That's why it is important to bring someone along for support during the first few
radiation sessions.

What happens during a radiotherapy session?

The radiation clinic will have a number of
radiation therapists on staff who will oper-
ate the machinery and administer your
treatment. You will go into a room that is
darkened when treatment starts and lie
down on something that looks like an examination table and has a device overhead
that activates the beam. You may then be
covered in lead blankets (this isn't always
done), and only the target area will be exposed. The beam will be turned on for a
maximum of three minutes—a completely
painless procedure. Your session will probably take about twenty minutes, however,
because it takes some time to re-position
the machine after the last patient and get
you in position for your treatment.

Figure 4.2
**BEING TATTOOED OR MARKED
FOR RADIATION THERAPY**

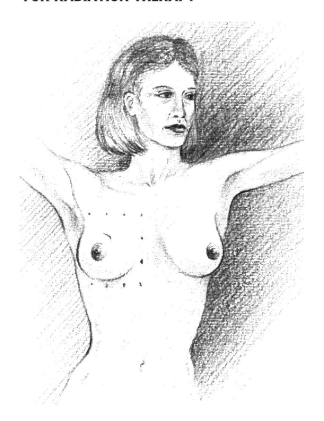

Dosage

Again, the amount of external radiation you will receive depends on the severity of your cancer. For example, you might only need thirty seconds of radiation
every weekday for a month, while another woman may require three minutes
of radiation every day for six weeks. The total dose of radiation you received is
measured in a unit called a Gray. The Grays are divided by the number of treatments you have received. This is called fractionation.

One Gray is equivalent to 100 rads. The average total dose of radiation in
breast cancer therapy ranges from 40 to 50 Grays (4,000 to 5,000 rads). A

woman who has, say, three weeks of radiation treatment (i.e., fifteen treatments altogether) will receive 2.6 Grays per treatment, assuming she has a total dose of 40 Grays. When you consider that the average mammogram delivers 0.0015 Grays, that's quite a bit. That's also why you may experience some side effects after radiotherapy.

Side effects

Although the radiation procedure itself is painless, the aftereffects are not. Knowing this in advance may not alleviate the symptoms, but it may make them more understandable, and therefore more bearable. Although radiation therapy today delivers far less radiation to tissues than even five years ago, you will still have side effects from the treatment. For the first week of treatment, you probably won't feel much. By week two, the squared-off area that the beam targeted will look and feel like a very bad sunburn. If you're fair-skinned, you'll probably have a worse reaction than people with darker pigment. A small raw area might develop in places where your skin rubs together—under the arms or beneath your breasts. Therefore, you will need to treat your skin as though it were sunburnt: avoid the sun, cover up exposed skin, don't use any deodorants or perfumes, use cornstarch and lotions safe for sunburnt or baby skin. Ask the radiation oncologist or radiation therapist on staff to recommend something that will help alleviate sunburn symptoms. Generally, diaper rash creams, or sunburn creams safe for babies are quite good. Creams that contain lanolin will soften and moisturize the burnt areas (such as Nivea cream, for example). If a small area of skin actually peels but has not become raw, a 1 percent cortisone cream helps. For itchiness, cornstarch in the bath or applied topically with a towel and bandage will help.

Your breasts may be very sore. You may find that the breast being irradiated becomes firmer than the other breast. It may enlarge and become tender and heavy with fluid for as long as six to eighteen months after treatment. You may also get little shocks of pain during and after treatment, which are caused by nerve endings trying to repair themselves, while little red burst blood vessels may appear anywhere from one to two years after treatment. You may find that going braless is best. Loose cotton clothing is recommended; wool can really irritate your breasts.

You'll also feel quite tired by the third or fourth week of treatment; the procedure is mentally as well as physically draining. You may experience some nausea (although this is rare with radiotherapy) or loss of appetite due to some of the other side effects. As soon as the treatments are finished, you'll start to feel much better and will regain your strength.

On rare occasions...

Most women will not require radiation beyond the breast areas. But sometimes it becomes necessary to expand the radiation field. If your upper chest or throat area is being radiated, your throat will feel extremely sore. You must absolutely not smoke during these treatments; smoking worsens the reactions in the throat and limits the effectiveness of the radiation. Swallowing may be very painful if your throat is irradiated, and as the treatment progresses, your throat may become so tender that you are better off spitting out your saliva than even attempting to swallow it. To relieve throat symptoms, the best thing to do is to continuously chew Aspergum. You can also request a topical anesthetic and/or analgesic, which numbs all feeling in your throat so you can eat. Obviously, eating soft and cold foods will be better. Or, if you are turned off to food altogether, you could survive on meal supplement drinks that are sold in drug stores and hospital pharmacies.

You may also experience a dry cough or sputum if the radiation is in your lung region. Cough suppressants should not be used because it is important to cough up the sputum. A humidifier will help to loosen the sputum so you can get rid of it.

Radiation in the chest region may also affect your esophageal region. Your esophagus is the long tube that connects your throat to your upper intestine, with a flap (the esophageal sphincter) that opens and closes as food goes down. Radiation can cause the esophagus to become inflamed, preventing the sphincter from closing properly after food is swallowed. The result is heartburn (where stomach acid escapes up into the esophagus, creating a burning sensation) and sometimes a feeling that the food is coming back up (known as reflux). There are a variety of acid suppressing medications available over the counter, such as Pepcid or Tagamet, which can alleviate these symptoms until your esophageal region heals.

Brachytherapy: "internal radiation"

This is sometimes given as a "booster" therapy after your external radiation therapy is over. Whether or not you will receive it depends on your oncologist's treatment philosophy and the extent of your cancer.

In this procedure, radiation oncologists plant a piece of radioactive material directly inside the tumor, or in the last known location of the tumor. In this case, a radioactive isotope (a radioactive element—as in the Table of Elements you had to memorize in science class), such as radioactive iridium, gold, or cesium, is used to "blast" the tumor from the inside out, rather than from the outside in as external radiation does. Tiny hollow tubes are surgically implanted into the targeted area (the tubes are later removed), and the isotopes are placed into the tubes on your treatment days. The side effects of internal radiation therapy will depend on the area in which isotopes are inserted. Some skin irritation in the treated areas is not uncommon, and is accompanied by loss of energy and appetite. Side effects *greatly* depend on what's being inserted where. You'll need to discuss this in more detail with your radiation oncologist and possibly a nuclear medicine specialist.

CHEMOTHERAPY

Chemotherapy was accidentally discovered when troops were exposed to mustard gas during both world wars. Although mustard gas wasn't officially used in World War II, it was during this war that the medicinal benefits of mustard gas became obvious. A ship carrying the gas was bombed in an Italian harbor. Survivors of the blast showed a dramatic drop in white blood cells—something that's bad news for healthy people, but good news for people with leukemia. The rest is history. Chemotherapy soon became standard treatment for leukemia, presenting the first possibility of a cure. Within a couple of decades, leukemia treatment became the basis for many cancer treatments, and poisonous agents began to be used to kill cancer cells.

Chemotherapy is standard treatment for all cancer patients. In other words, chemotherapy for ovarian cancer, leukemia, or breast cancer is the same. This treatment is by far the most miserable, and for many women, it makes the notion of having cancer a reality. In the past, chemotherapy was reserved for cases where surgery had failed to treat the cancer. Today, even when there is no sign of cancer after surgery, chemotherapy can be used as a preventive or pro-phylactic therapy, known as adjuvant chemotherapy.

What exactly is chemotherapy?

Chemotherapy simply means treating a medical condition with drugs. So, tech-nically, taking aspirin or an antibiotic is a form of chemotherapy. When it comes to cancer, chemotherapy involves taking anticancer drugs. These drugs are de-signed to kill cancer cells, which they do by interfering with the process of cell division or reproduction so that cancer cells can't divide and therefore die. But the drugs are not very selective and they kill healthy cells that are also dividing, including hair cells and bone marrow cells.

Basically the line between a therapeutic dosage and a toxic dosage is quite fine, which is why only a highly experienced medical oncologist is qualified to manage your chemotherapy. Chemotherapy drugs can be administered orally or intravenously. You might be given just one drug, or a combination of drugs. Combination drug therapy is often done because most chemotherapy drugs are not selective as far as cancer cells are concerned, so multiple drugs are used to overcome drug resistance.

Who is a chemo candidate?

If there is no evidence that your cancer has spread and the tumor was small and localized, or in situ, you won't be offered chemotherapy. You probably won't be offered chemotherapy if you're over sixty-five either, unless your cancer is quite advanced, or node positive and estrogen-receptor and progesterone-receptor negative. Chemotherapy is hard on the body, and generally doesn't do an older body any good unless there's a really high probability of the cancer recurring.

Chemotherapy is recommended if you find yourself in one or more of the following scenarios:

1. Your cancer has spread to the axillary lymph nodes (lymph nodes under the arm) and you're premenopausal. (This means your ovaries are still making estrogen, which, chances are, the cancer thrives on).
2. Your lymph nodes are negative, but your tumor was larger than a centimeter in diameter (tumors that are 1 to 2 cm in diameter are considered larger).
3. There is evidence that your cancer has spread into the nerves or the lymphatic or vascular channels of the breast.
4. While there is no clear evidence your cancer has spread, you're in a high-risk group for recurrence.

Common anti-cancer drugs

Once you enter the world of cancer drugs, you can become overwhelmed by the various names of drugs. One doctor may refer to a drug by its brand name, while another doctor may use its generic name. For clarity, the generic name appears first in the following paragraph, while a common brand name is in parentheses—as in ibuprofen (Advil) and acetaminophen (Tylenol). Also review table 4.1.

Drugs you may come across during your treatment include doxorubicin (Adriamycin); cyclophosphamide (Cytoxan); fluorouracil (Adrucil), which has another generic name—5-fluorouracil, nicknamed "5-FU"; methotrexate sodium (Methotrexate); and epirubicin hydrochloride (Pharmorubicin). Occasionally, vincristine sulfate (Oncovin) and prednisone (no specific brand name associated with this drug) are used as well.

When you're given these drugs in combination, the therapy is referred to by the acronym that forms when you put the generic names together. The only drug that is ever referred to by brand name within such acronyms is

Adriamycin. In other words, the "A" in *any* chemo acronym stands for Adriamycin. So for example, AC means your therapy is a combination of Adriamycin and cyclophosphamide. CMF means you're getting cyclophosphamide, methotrexate, and 5-FU. CAF would mean cyclophosphamide, Adriamycin, and 5-FU. CEF refers to cyclophosphamide, epirubicin, and 5-FU.

Possible contraindications

Chemotherapy drugs are very powerful drugs. As a result, some of you may not be able to take certain chemotherapy drugs if you have any "contraindicated" conditions—which may have nothing to do with your cancer.

Although medical oncologists take detailed medical histories so they can prescribe the chemo regimen that best suits your physique, it is important to be aware of the following facts (and let your doctor know, too):

1. You cannot have chemotherapy if you are in the early stages of pregnancy, although most drugs can be administered after the first trimester. Get a pregnancy test first, so you know.
2. You may not be able to have chemotherapy if you have chronic liver disease (especially if it is caused by alcoholism). You need a good, healthy liver to metabolize the drugs.
3. You may not be able to have certain drugs if you are already immunodeficient from HIV or a previous course of chemotherapy. You need to start with a healthy white blood cell count. (This is discussed further on.)
4. Since certain chemo drugs can induce lung disease, you shouldn't start chemotherapy if you have a pre-existing pulmonary disorder.
5. *Always* check with your medical oncologist before you take any over-the-counter drugs or prescription medications. Painkillers that fall into the non-steroidal anti-inflammatory (NSAIDs) or salicylates categories are especially dangerous. Certain antibiotics can also reduce or increase the effectiveness of your chemotherapy.
6. Certain drugs may not be able to be administered if you have a pre-existing kidney disorder (although many of these drugs will affect your kidney function temporarily).

Table 4.1

TWENTY-TWO COMMONLY USED ANTI-CANCER DRUGS

Aminoglutethimide, brand name Cytadren. An antihormonal agent, administered orally. Used to treat breast, prostate, and adrenal cancer. More common side effects include clumsiness, dizziness or lightheadedness when standing up, drowsiness, lack of energy, loss of appetite, skin rash or itching, nausea, and uncontrolled eye movements.

Androgens, generic names include fluoxymesterone, methyitestosterone, testosterone, testosterone cypionate, testosterone enanthate, and testosterone propionate. More than forty brand names exist for the androgens, so check with your pharmacist, doctor, or nurse for the name of your drug. Androgens are male hormones, administered orally. Used to treat breast cancer in females, and for some other conditions. For females, the most common side effects, which should be reported to your doctor, include acne or oily skin, enlarged clitoris, hair loss, deepening of voice, irregular periods, and unnatural hair growth. For males, the most com-

mon side effects, which should be reported to your doctor, include acne, breast soreness, frequent erections, frequent urge to urinate, and increased breast size.

Cyclophosphamide, brand names include Cytoxan and NEOSAR. An alkylating agent, administered orally or by injection. Used to treat some types of cancer including Hodgkin's and non-Hodgkin's lymphoma, multiple myeloma, sarcomas, leukemia, neuroblastoma, breast, lung, testes, endometrium, mycosis fungoides cancer, and kidney disease. Side effects, which should be reported to your doctor, include dizziness, confusion or agitation, unusual fatigue, and missing menstrual periods. More common side effects include bone marrow suppression, hair loss, darkening of skin or fingernails, loss of appetite, nausea, and vomiting.

Doxorubicin, or Adriamycin PFS, Adriamycin RDF, or Rubex. An antitumor antibiotic, administered by injection. Used to treat

some types of cancers including lung, breast, bladder, prostate, pancreas, stomach, ovary, thyroid, endometrium, sarcoma, leukemia, Hodgkin's and non-Hodgkin's lymphoma, mesothelioma myeloma, Wilms' tumor and cancer of unknown primary site. Side effects, which should be reported to your doctor, include sores in mouth or on lips. Most common side effects include nausea and vomiting and loss of hair. Urine will turn red in color for one to two days after treatment.

Estradiol, or Estraderm. A hormonal agent, administered through patches placed on the skin. Provides additional hormones after certain types of surgery in females, and for other conditions. Side effects, which should be reported to your doctor, include breast pain, increased breast size, swelling of feet or lower legs, and rapid weight gain. More common side effects include bloating of stomach, cramps, loss of appetite, nausea, skin irritation, and redness on site of patch.

Table 4.1 *continued*

Estrogens (IV). Generic names include chlorotrianisene, diethylstilbestrol, estradiol, estrogens, estrone, estropipate, ethinyl estradiol, and quinestrol. More than sixty brand names exist for estrogens—consult your pharmacist, doctor, or nurse for the name of your drug. A female hormone, administered by injection. Used to treat some cases of breast cancer in men or women, prostate cancer, to provide additional hormones after surgery, and for other conditions. Side effects, which should be reported to your doctor, include breast pain, increased breast size, and swelling of feet and lower legs. Another side effect for women who have not had their uterus removed and are taking estrogen in combination with the female hormone progestin is that they may begin having monthly vaginal bleeding similar to menstruation.

Estrogens (oral). More than sixty brand names and generic names (see number 21). A female hormone, administered orally. Used to treat some cases of breast cancer in men or women, prostate cancer, to provide additional hormones after surgery, and for other conditions. Side effects are similar to estrogens in number 21, with the addition of nausea and vomiting, which are more common.

Fluorouracil, or Adrucil or 5-FU. An antimetabolite, administered by injection. Used to treat some types of cancer including breast, stomach, colon, liver, pancreas, ovarian, bladder, and prostate cancer. Can be used topically for skin cancer. Side effects, which should be reported to your doctor immediately, include diarrhea, heartburn, and sores in mouth and on lips. More common side effects include bone marrow suppression, loss of appetite, nausea and vomiting, skin rash or itching, loss of hair, and fatigue.

Goserelin, or Zoladex. A hormonal agent, administered by injection. Used in some cases of prostate cancer. More common side effects include decrease in sexual desire, impotence, and sudden sweating or hot flashes.

Leucovorin, or Wellcovorin, folinic acid, citrovorum factor, or leucovorin calcium. A protecting agent, administered orally or by injection. Used as an antidote to some anticancer drugs such as methotrexate, or a potentiating agent when used with fluorouracil. Also prevents or treats certain types of anemia. Side effects, which should be reported to your doctor immediately, include skin rash, hives, itching, and wheezing.

Leuprolide, or Lupron or Lupron Depot. A hormonal agent, administered by injection. Used to treat cancer of the prostate, and for other conditions. More common side effects include decrease in sexual desire or impotence, nausea or vomiting, and sudden sweats or hot flashes.

Table 4.1 continued

TWENTY-TWO COMMONLY USED ANTI-CANCER DRUGS

Methotrexate, or Folex, Folex PFS, Mexate, Mexate-AQ, Rheumatrex, or amethopterin. An antimetabolite, administered orally or by injection. Used to treat some types of cancer including acute leukemia, sarcoma, choriocarcinoma, head and neck, breast, lung, stomach, esophagus, testes, lymphoma, and mycosis fungoides. Side effects, which should be reported to your doctor immediately, include black, tarry stools, bloody vomit, diarrhea, reddening of skin, sores in mouth or on lips, and stomach pain. Most common side effects include bone marrow suppression, nausea, and vomiting.

Mitomycin, or Mutamycin. An alkylating agent, administered by injection. Used to treat some types of cancers including colon, stomach, pancreas, esophagus, anus, breast, lung, cervix, and bladder cancer. Most common side effects include bone marrow suppression, nausea, vomiting, loss of appetite, and sometimes loss of hair.

Mitoxantrone, or Novantrone. An antitumor antibiotic, administered by injection. Used to treat some types of cancer in-

cluding acute leukemia, breast, ovarian, and lymphomas. Side effects, which should be reported to your doctor immediately, include black, tarry stools, coughing, and shortness of breath. Another side effect, which should be reported to your doctor, is stomach pain. More common side effects include diarrhea, headaches, nausea, and vomiting.

Prednisone, or Apr-Prednisone, Deltasone, Liquid Pred, Meticorten, Orasone 1, Orasone 5, Orasone 10, Orasone 20, Orasone 50, Prednicen-M, Prednisone Intensol, Sterapred, Sterapred DS, or Winpred. An adrenocorticoid or hormonal agent which is administered orally. Used to treat acute and chronic lymphocytic leukemia, Hodgkin's and non-Hodgkin's lymphoma, myeloma, breast, and brain metastases, as well as some noncancerous conditions. Common side effects include increased appetite, indigestion, nervousness, restlessness, and trouble sleeping. Side effects, which should be reported to your doctor with long-term use, include back or rib pain, bloody or black stools, chronic stomach pain or burning, puffiness in face, irregular heartbeats, menstrual problems,

muscle cramps, pain, fatigue, reddish purple lines on skin, swelling of feet, thin or shiny skin, and rapid weight gain.

Progestins, or progestinal agents, known by several other names including Amen, Aygestin, Curretab, Cycrin, Delalutin, Depo-Provera, Duralutin, Femotrone, Gesterol L.A., Hylutin, Hyprogest, Hyproval P.A., Megace, Micronor, Norethisterone, Norlutate, Norlutin, Nor-QD, Ovrette, Pro-Depo, Prodrox, Progestaject, Progestilin, and Provera. A hormonal agent, administered orally. Used to treat breast, prostate, uterine, and kidney cancer. These side effects are rare with this drug, but you should immediately get emergency help if you experience a sudden or severe headache, loss of coordination, loss or change in vision, shortness of breath or slurred speech, pains in chest, groin, or leg, unusual weakness, numbness, and pain in arm or leg. A more common side effect is a change in the menstrual cycle, which should be reported to your doctor. More common side effects include changes in appetite, changes in weight, swelling of ankles and feet, unusual tiredness, and weakness.

Table 4.1 continued

Tamoxifen, or Nolvadex, Novadex-D, or tamoxifen citrate. An antihormonal agent, administered orally. Used to treat some cases of breast cancer, endometrium, and ovarian cancer. More common side effects include hot flashes, nausea or vomiting, and weight gain.

Taxol, or Paclitaxel. An antineoplastic, administered by injectionl. Used to treat cancers such as cancer of the breast or ovary. Side effects, which should be reported to your doctor immediately, include cough or harshness, fever or chills, lower back or side pain, and painful or difficult urination. More common side effects, which should also be reported to your doctor, include flushing of face, shortness of breath, and skin rash or itching. Other common side effects your doctor will watch for include anemia and low white blood cell or platelet counts. Other more common side effects include diarrhea, nausea and vomiting, numbness, burning, tingling in hands or feet,

and pain in joints or muscles such as arms or legs beginning two to three days after treatment, which can last as long as five days.

Testolactone, or Teslac. A hormonal agent, administered orally. Used to treat some cases of breast cancer in females. Infrequently causes diarrhea, loss of appetite, nausea or vomiting, pain in lower extremities, rash, and swelling or redness of tongue.

Thiotepa, or triethylenethiophosphoramide. An alkylating agent, administered by injection. Used to treat some types of cancer such as breast, bladder, ovarian, Hodgkin's disease, and bone marrow transplantation. Most common side effect is bone marrow suppression.

Vinblastine, or Velban, Velsar, or vinblastine sulfate. A plant alkaloid, administered by injection. Used to treat some types of cancer such as Hodgkin's disease, choriocarcinoma, testes, breast,

lung, and Kaposi's sarcoma. Most common side effects include bone marrow suppression, nausea, vomiting, constipation, and sometimes loss of hair. Can cause burns if it leaks out of the vein.

Vincristine, or Oncovin, Vincasar PFS, Vincrez, or vincristine sulfate. A plant alkaloid, administered by injection. Used to treat some types of cancer including acute lymphocytic leukemia, Hodgkin's and non-Hodgkin's lymphoma, neuroblastoma, testes, sarcomas, lung, breast, cervical cancer, and Wilms' tumor. Side effects, which should be reported to your doctor, include blurred or double vision, constipation, difficulty walking, drooping eyelids, headache, jaw pain, joint pain, lower back or side pain, numbness or tingling in fingers and toes, pain in fingers and toes, pain in testicles, stomach cramps, swelling of feet or lower legs, and weakness. Can cause loss of hair.

Source: Drum, David, Making the Chemotherapy Decision, Los Angeles: Lowell House, 1996, 96–109.

7. Let your doctor know about any bacterial, fungal, or viral infection. Insist on a full pelvic exam prior to chemotherapy so you can be screened for vaginal infections (yeast or bacterial vaginosis) as well as sexually transmitted diseases (many are asymptomatic). Chicken pox or shingles (varicella) can be especially problematic with certain drugs. You may have been exposed through your children.

8. If you are on hormone replacement therapy (HRT) or on any kind of hormonal contraceptive, you must stop before beginning chemotherapy.

9. If you have a pre-existing cardiac problem, you should not be on certain chemo drugs.

10. If you wear an IUD (intrauterine device), have it removed before starting chemotherapy. Some drugs can cause inflammation of the uterine lining, which can severely aggravate an IUD.

Dosage

If you've ever been on a birth control pill, you will be familiar with having drugs in cycles. That is exactly how chemotherapy is administered. Some chemotherapy works on a 21- or 28-day cycle—various oral and intravenous drugs are administered for the first two weeks, followed by a drug-free rest period. This is dubbed by insiders as the "two weeks on/two weeks off" cycle. You may also be given a variety of drugs for the first five days, followed by a 21-day rest period. Dosages vary from person to person. They depend on your overall health prior to the chemo, the extent of your cancer, and a hundred other factors. Many of the side effects discussed next can be signs of over- or underdosing; the dose will need to be adjusted as your course of therapy continues.

How many weeks are we talking about?

Chemotherapy regimens last anywhere from three to six months. In more advanced cases of breast cancer, you will have a course of chemo, then a wait-and-see period, which is sometimes followed by a repeat course of treatment.

It is possible to have a recurrence, discussed in Chapter 8, after being cancer-free for years. If you have a recurrence, you may need to repeat chemotherapy for the other breast.

Cancer cells have a nasty habit of developing resistance to chemotherapy drugs by increasing the levels of a cell membrane molecule called glocosylceramide, similar to bacteria that can resist antiobiotics. Tamoxifen, verapamil, and cyclosporin A seem to be able to inhibit glucosylceramide from forming. Nevertheless, drug resistance is the major obstacle to a successful bout with chemotherapy.

The general side effects

Each drug comes with its own list of potential side effects. For example, epirubicin will turn your urine red; while doxirubicin can increase your risk of heart disease. Since space doesn't allow me to list the side effects for every drug or combination of drugs (this is enough information for a separate book), it is important to research each specific drug you are taking. Pharmacists recommend getting information from the United States Pharmacopeia Drug Information (USPDI) or the American Society of Hospital Pharmacists' book of drug information for consumers. Many pharmacies now offer extensive drug information for patients as an added service. Another option is to look up your drug in a pharmaceutical compendium, such as the Physician's Desk Reference (available in libraries), for the complete story—this information is very technical, however, and may not be suitable for the layperson. At any rate, I recommend getting the information before you start your drug therapy so you can review it with your doctor and be fully prepared for the side effects of the drugs, among other things.

You will find during your research that there are general side effects that are common to all anti-cancer drugs. That's because no matter how balanced your chemotherapy dosage is, healthy cells will be affected. Reactions do vary from person to person, however, and there are certain medications such as anti-nausea drugs (Zofran is a common one) that are often added to the therapy to reduce the infamous vomiting and nausea.

Some of the more common reactions to chemo include: tiredness, weakness, body aches, bloating and weight gain, night sweats, nausea, loss of appetite, and a change in your sense of taste and smell (you may notice a chemical odor all the time, for instance). It's not uncommon to have mouth sores, dry mouth, pink eye (conjunctivitis), "allergy symptoms" (watery eyes and runny nose), bleeding gums, and headaches, as well as diarrhea and constipation. Less common are tingling fingers and toes and loss of muscle strength. These reactions can be mild, moderate, or severe; and medications can relieve many of the symptoms.

Believe it or not, monosodium glutamate (MSG) has been shown to prevent some of the side effects of anti-cancer drugs. It may help prevent nerve damage, which affects about one-fifth of all people being treated for breast cancer. In short, a little Chinese food may go a long way to improve cure rates with chemotherapy, enabling more intensive chemotherapy to be administered over longer periods of time.

Chemo can also cause a chemically induced depression (charmingly known as "chemo brain") and dramatic mood swings. If you're menstruating, your periods will become irregular, or they may stop altogether. This happens because your ovaries begin to fail, causing surgical menopause, discussed further on (although not every woman will experience surgical menopause).

Now for the most disturbing side effect: hair loss (clinically known as alopecia). First, it is important to be prepared for hair loss, but there is also a possibility that your hair may *not* fall out. For most women, the idea of losing hair is worse than actually losing it; hair loss is a loss of femininity and an announcement to the world that you have cancer. Talking to a counselor and sharing your feelings with other chemo patients will help put this side effect in perspective. Some women's hair may thin gradually, while other women may find that they lose their hair all of sudden. Still others may find that it comes out in clumps. Whatever your experience, if you do lose your hair, you'll begin to notice it three or four weeks into your treatment. You will also lose all other hair on your body: pubic hair, leg hair (you might hope *this* is permanent), eyebrows, eyelashes, and so on.

One way to get around this side effect is to find a good wig before your chemotherapy and have your hairdresser style it like your current hairstyle. That way, the wig won't look obvious, and your hair loss will not be as apparent. Many women simply wear scarves, hats, or turbans.

Other side effects include a decrease in blood platelets, which are responsible for blood clotting. You might find that you're bruising easily, that you bleed more when you're cut, or bleed suddenly out of your nose or even rectum. This will get better after your treatment, but please report your bleeding episodes to your doctor so your dosage can be adjusted if necessary.

After your treatment is over, you will slowly start to feel better. You will gradually regain your old energy and the depression will lift. In most cases, hair does grow back, although, the new hair might be a different texture (curly, if you had straight hair before, or vice versa) or a different color (black to gray). You will also shed the bloating and your complexion will return to normal. Food will taste right again, and you may crave foods you never craved in the past. You *will* be yourself once again.

A word about surgical menopause

When your body goes into menopause as a result of the surgical removal of your ovaries (oopherectomy) or because your ovaries have become sterilized due to drugs or radiation to the pelvic area, this is known as surgical menopause. (Natural menopause occurs when the body naturally uses up its eggs without any outside interference.)

Surgical menopause may be a gradual process; more often, though, women are overwhelmed by the suddenness of the symptoms. The speed at which menopause sets in depends on the kind of therapy you've received and the speed at which the ovaries are failing. Before you undergo cancer treatment, ask the doctor how the treatments will affect your ovaries and what menopausal symptoms you can expect.

The first sign of surgical menopause is erratic periods. Intervals between menstrual cycles may become longer or shorter; flow may become heavier or lighter, until, eventually, the periods taper off altogether. You will begin to notice the classic symptoms of estrogen loss, including vaginal dryness and hot flashes.

Vaginal dryness will cause some sexual discomfort, which can be relieved with lubricants.

A hot flash can feel different to each woman. Some women experience a feeling of warmth in their face and upper body; some experience hot flashes as simultaneous sweating and chills. Some women feel anxious, tense, dizzy, or nauseous just before the hot flash; some feel tingling in their fingers or heart palpitations just before. Some women will experience their hot flashes during the day; others will experience them at night and may wake up so wet from perspiration that they need to change their bedsheets and/or night clothes. Nobody really understands what causes a hot flash, but researchers believe that it has to do with mixed signals from the hypothalamus, which controls both body temperature and sex hormones.

Hormone replacement therapy (HRT)—not to be confused with hormone therapy for breast cancer—can relieve menopause symptoms, but you may *not* be able to have HRT if your breast cancer is thought to thrive on estrogen. Nor should you be on hormone replacement therapy while you are undergoing chemotherapy, as discussed in the chemotherapy contraindications section.

Warning signs

If you experience any of the following symptoms, notify your doctor immediately—it may be a sign that you need to stop the chemotherapy immediately.

1. Severe diarrhea.
2. Severe stomach pains (sign of gastritis—inflammation of your stomach lining).
3. Dry cough (without sputum or mucus)—sign of a possible lung infection.
4. An active infection or virus (flu-like symptoms and fever should be reported).
5. Fever (especially if accompanied by a dry cough).
6. Shortness of breath.
7. Painful, frequent urination. (Symptom of a urinary tract infection, which could be an early sign of bladder inflammation).

Many of these alarm symptoms occur if the dosage is too high. The general practice is to modify the chemo dosage at the next cycle.

About your white blood cells...

All blood cells and platelets are made inside the bone marrow. Normally, the bone marrow will be able to recover from the chemotherapy and bring your counts back to normal. But one definite warning sign that your chemotherapy may need to be stopped for a while is a dangerously low white blood cell count (WBC). This is something you can't notice yourself (flu-like fatigue is a symptom, but you wouldn't realize that), but it will be apparent in your lab reports. If this is the case, your dosage should be adjusted or chemotherapy should be delayed until your white blood cell count comes back up.

Sometimes women are given a white blood cell growth hormone called granulocyte cell stimulating factor (GCSF). This hormone stimulates your body to superproduce white blood cells, raising your count dramatically (from, say, 10,000 to 50,000) so your chemotherapy can be continued.

But what happens when a very high-dose chemotherapy regimen is necessary in some cases of advanced breast cancer? In such cases, something known as a stem cell transplant is done before the next chemotherapy regimen.

To understand what a stem cell transplant is, think about what happens in an in vitro fertilization procedure. A woman is given fertility drugs to help her ovaries grow eggs. These eggs are then "rescued" from the ovaries and placed in a petri dish. Same thing happens here, except that instead of fertility drugs, you are given the GCFS hormone. The hormone helps the growth of white blood cells—the stem cells. These stem cells are rescued through an intravenous procedure. Blood is taken out of one arm and passed back into the other arm, and while this is happening, your stem cells are "caught" in midstream and saved in bags. After your high-dose chemotherapy, the stem cells are returned to you intravenously. The stem cells then start producing white blood cells, but this can take some time. Meanwhile, your white blood cell count can plummet to almost zero. This will make you feel awful, like you were hit with a supermegaflu, and you will need to be kept in isolation during your chemo regimen. You will also need to be careful about exposure to infections and bacteria, since your immune system will be completely suppressed.

Long-term risks

Because chemotherapy blasts the hell out of your white blood cells, it increases your risk of developing leukemia and other kinds of cancers. This risk is, thankfully, low compared to the benefits you receive from chemotherapy.

Your risk of other diseases such as heart disease and lung or liver disorders can also increase due to the potency of the drugs used. Again, the benefits usually outweigh the risk, but you should discuss all potential long-term risks with your doctor before you begin your therapy.

Finally, many of you will be in surgical menopause by the end of your chemo, which brings all the risks associated with estrogen-loss into the picture: heart disease and osteoporosis, accompanied by more short-term symptoms, such as vaginal dryness and hot flashes.

HORMONE THERAPY

Hormone therapy (sometimes called endocrine therapy) may be offered to you if your cancer is more advanced and estrogen-receptor positive or progesterone-receptor positive (this means that the hormones estrogen and/or progesterone help the cancer cells to grow). A hormone receptor is the lock; the hormone itself is the key. If a breast cancer is estrogen-receptor positive (ER-positive), for example, it means that the breast cancer cells have little "keys" that can fit into this lock. In order to find out whether the cancer is estrogen- or progesteroune-receptor positive, a piece of the tumor that was removed during surgery is tested with a chemical that can measure how many, if any, estrogen or progesterone receptors there are on the cancer cell.

The theory behind hormone therapy is this: If female hormones make breast cancer grow, we can stop breast cancer by removing female hormones from the body.

It is a little difficult to just remove female hormones from the body, of course. There are basically three routes available to your medical practitioners. One route is to surgically remove your ovaries, which will put you into surgical menopause (see page 148) if you're premenopausal. Another route is to deaden your ovaries with drugs (chemotherapy) or with radiation to the pelvic area. The third, and most popular, route is to somehow block estrogen and/or progesterone with drugs. The drugs you're offered depend on your age.

Drugs for premenopausal women

If you've read Chapter 10 (pages 265–268), you already know that tamoxifen is anti-estrogen (a.k.a. estrogen blocker). And you also know about the contentious issues involved with using tamoxifen as a prevention therapy. But when it comes to treating breast cancer, tamoxifen is generally offered to postmenopausal women only, because that is the group in which it has proven to be effective 30 to 35 percent of the time, compared to a dismal 12 percent efficacy in premenopausal women. Researchers believe that in premenopausal women the ovaries interfere with the anti-estrogenic effect of tamoxifen.

Therefore, another drug called goserelin (Zoladex) is used for premenopausal women. Goserelin inhibits hormone production at the hormonal "head office": the pituitary gland. In the case of premenopausal women with breast cancer, goserelin stops the production of *luteinizing hormone*, which eggs need to make estrogen. Goserelin is therefore used not only in cases of advanced breast cancer in premenopausal women, but in women suffering from endometriosis, as well as in men with prostate cancer (goserelin also prevents the testes from producing testosterone). Women on goserelin will have the same estrogen levels as postmenopausal women.

Goserelin has a number of side effects. Many of the side effects of goserelin are menopause-type symptoms, linked to a decrease in estrogen. These include hot flashes, vaginal dryness, and decreased libido. But goserelin's side effects also include joint pain, bone pain, headaches, depression, dry mouth, nausea, rashes, and a host of other problems. By the way, you cannot be on goserelin if you've had any vaginal bleeding (unless your doctor has checked it out). You must not be pregnant or lactating while on this medication, either, nor can you be on any other hormonal contraceptive. Always rule out a pregnancy before you begin this therapy.

Premenopausal women are usually given hormone therapy for *advanced* breast cancer. In advanced cases, the cancer has spread to other parts of the body and has graduated to metastatic disease, discussed in Chapter 8.

When cancer has mestastized, progestins are also used to counteract the effects of estrogen in the body. Megestrol acetate (Megace) is a common progestin that has about a 30 percent response rate overall (including both pre- and postmenopausal women). If you've ever taken the "mini-pill" (a progestin-only birth control pill) or a combination oral contraceptive, you can expect a repeat of the identical side effects, including weight gain and breakthrough bleeding, which are common complaints, although hot flashes have also been reported. Weight gain is the result of the huge increase in appetite that is another nuisance side effect of megestrol. The appetite increase is so great on this drug that its use is being considered in certain illnesses where weight loss is a problem.

Drugs for postmenopausal women

Tamoxifen is the "Coke Classic" of hormone therapies for estrogen-receptor positive tumors in postmenopausal women. But even in this group, tamoxifen has a success rate of 35 percent at best.

Since the introduction of tamoxifen in the 1980s, hormone therapy has been undergoing some fine-tuning. Tamoxifen can be considered a cruder version of new drugs that are trying to target hormone receptors more effectively and with less severe side effects. Unfortunately, new formulations take time to develop and get approval.

A newer drug in the postmenopausal age group is the *aromatase inhibitor.* Aromatase is an enzyme that helps to convert estrogen from hormones secreted by the adrenal gland. This enzyme is found in muscle, fat, and the liver (this is how estrogen is made from fat). Aromatase inhibitors seem to have a promising future in treating breast cancer and a lower side effect profile.

Dosages

Dosages on hormone therapy drugs really vary. They depend on your age, the stage of your cancer, and the drugs themselves. All these drugs are given in pill form. A typical dose of tamoxifen varies from 20 to 40 mg daily for a duration of two to five years.

NOW WHAT?

A breast cancer patient is an outpatient for the rest of her life. But there is now considerable literature in the medical community about the value of regimented, regular follow-ups over simply going for a follow-up visit when you feel like it or need to.

Depending on the philosophy of your specialist regarding this issue, you may still be going for regular visits to all your cancer doctors: medical and radiation oncologists and/or breast surgeon and/or gynecologic oncologist. Each specialist may see you every three months for the first two years; then every six months for the next four or five years; and then, annually. Each visit will entail various diagnostic tests: blood tests, chest X rays, bone scans, CAT scans, mammograms.

The ultimate question is: are you cured after all these treatments? The answer depends on the stage your cancer was in to begin with (see Chapter 3). Statistically, the answer is "usually."

Cancer goes into remission, meaning that the cells stop growing and what *was* there was removed or effectively killed. But cancer cells can start up again and begin to grow at some future point. Sometimes the recurrence is local; sometimes the recurrence takes place elsewhere in your body (known as metastatic disease: "spread disease"). This is especially true of breast cancer, which is why follow-ups are so important. If you've had a mastectomy or wide excision, it is crucial to have a mammogram done on both breasts regularly. You should also be performing breast self-exams monthly (see table 4.2 for postsurgical exams). Usually, the longer you are cancer-free, the greater your chances of being permanently cured. But there are women who have recurrences a decade after their first bout with breast cancer. Everything you need to know about recurrence and metastatic disease is discussed in Chapter 8.

HEY—WHAT ABOUT MY HEALTH INSURANCE?

Since the insurance industry is regulated by state, check with your state's insurance commission about what's specifically available. Most companies with at least twenty-five employees offer group medical insurance that has good, affordable coverage. Most of these policies have a "pre-existing condition" clause which means that if you start a new job after you've been diagnosed with breast cancer, you may not be covered for any breast cancer-related treatment for up to 12 months. After 12 months, however, coverage for breast cancer would resume.

1. Don't let your insurance lapse. Your present insurer can't drop your policy because of breast cancer, but if the policy lapses, it might be hard to find a new insurer after you have been ill. Any government-funded insurance severely limits your medical care choices, so be sure to pay the premiums of your current plan.

2. If you're changing jobs, make sure you can transfer your insurance from one job to the next. Or, make sure your next employer has a good health plan before you discontinue any existing coverage. Keep in mind that under the COBRA law, you're entitled to continued coverage under your group health insurance plan if you leave your job for some reason. But you have to pay the cost of your group coverage as well as the administrative fee to your former employer to stay on the plan. You must also give your employer appropriate notice that you want to continue your coverage (notice period varies by plan). If your continuation coverage does run out, you may be entitled to extending benefits; check!

3. If you've left your job because of your illness, make every effort to pay the premiums yourself so you can keep the policy alive—even if you need to borrow the money.

4. If you're unemployed or your employer does not offer medical insurance, several professional groups and social organizations offer group insurance plans. These are usually more expensive, but it's better than government insurance and better than nothing.

5. After you've been diagnosed with breast cancer, you will not be eligible for most individual insurance plans with commercial insurance companies. But, if you already have a policy, it cannot be changed or canceled as a result of your breast cancer. You can still buy individual insurance in several states through the Blue Cross/Blue Shield open-enrollment program. These policies aren't wonderful and have some truly limiting

Table 4.2

HOW TO DO BSE AFTER A MASTECTOMY

If you continue to menstruate, the best time to do BSE is seven to ten days after the first day of your cycle. This is the time during your menstrual cycle when the breast is least tender to touch. Remember, if you had premenstrual breast tenderness before your mastectomy, you will probably continue to feel that discomfort in your remaining breast. Discomfort that comes and goes with your period is not a sign of breast cancer. If you no longer menstruate, pick a day, such as the first day of the month, to do BSE.

A breast examination has two parts, the visual exam and the palpation (touch) exam. During the visual examination, you will look at yourself in a mirror. During the palpation exam, you will use your hand to examine yourself. If you find any changes, show them to your doctors.

The Visual Examination

Stand in front of a mirror. Hold your hands (palm side down) in front of you. Compare your unaffected hand to your affected. Notice if you have any swelling in your affected hand. Then with your arms at your side, look in the mirror and compare the size of your arms. Do you notice any swelling? If so, you may be developing lymphedema and should make an appointment to begin treatment.

Next, with arms at your side, stand and examine your whole chest area from your collarbone to your bra line, and from the middle of your chest to your underarm area.

Raise your hands above your head. Slowly, turn from side to side, so that you can examine from the middle of your chest to your underarm area. If you notice any of the following changes, show them to your doctor:

- Persistent rash, redness, or discoloration of your scar, chest, and/or breast.
- Persistent itchy rash on your nipple or areola.
- Nipple discharge that is spontaneous and persistent.
- A change in the size or shape of your breast, such as a dimple.
- A lump in your scar, chest, and/or breast.

The Palpation Examination

During the palpation examination, you will use your hands to examine yourself.

Lie on your back and use your opposite hand to examine yourself. For example, if you are examining your right side, use your left hand.

If your breast size is B cup or large, the following position will spread your breast tissue evenly over your chest. Turn on your side with your knees bent, as if you were going to sleep on your side; then turn your upper body away from you bent knees, so that your chest faces the ceiling.

Hold your hand flat and use the fleshy pads of your middle three fingers, rather than the tips.

At each spot you examine, move the pads of your fingers in three small circles–about the size of a dime. Use three levels of pressure–light, medium, and deep. When pressing deeply, try to feel your ribs. Your ribs feel like a washboard.

A good examination pattern is the "vertical strip method." Always start in your armpit and examine down toward your bra line.

When you examine the side of your mastectomy, pay particular attention to your scar. If you notice a hard lump, a thickening, or any change, show it to your doctor.

Source: Benedet, Rosalind Dolores, N.P., M.S.N. Healing: A Woman's Guide to Recovery after Mastectomy. San Francisco: R. Benedet Publishing, 1993: 69–73.

clauses, but again, they may be better than nothing. Check with your local Blue Cross/Blue Shield office for details.

6. If you're really stuck, there are state-sponsored "high-risk" pools. This coverage is pretty expensive, but may be your only option. And if medical expenses are really high, a few states sponsor what's called catastrophic health insurance programs. Again, this is outrageously expensive, but may be your only hope.

7. Medicare is a U.S. federally funded program that pays partial costs for people who: are 65-years-old and over; have permanent kidney failure; or have been eligible for Social Security Disability Insurance (SSDI) benefits for two years.

8. Medicaid is a local, state, and federally funded program that covers health care expenses for some people without medical insurance, provided that their income levels are below the poverty line. If you're already receiving Social Security Disability Insurance or Aid to Families with Dependent Children (AFDC), you automatically qualify for Medicaid. If you have no insurance and any money in the bank, you're expected to completely exhaust that money before you qualify. Some people have tried transferring their savings to a friend's account. Transfers of large sums are usually checked and this trick doesn't work anymore.

9. If you're battling end-stage cancer (see Chapter 9), and you've exhausted your savings and have no insurance coverage anymore, you can look into collecting on your life insurance policy right now. This used to be impossible, but thanks to many AIDS activists, it's being done more and more. Check with your life insurer to see if you qualify. See the back of the book under "Finances and Insurance" for numbers to call.

· · · · · · ·

For many of you, the worst is over and the living can begin again. For a lot of women, getting back to life may involve not just an inner period of reconstruction, but actual reconstructive surgery. The next chapter discusses all your reconstructive options, as well as alternatives to reconstructive surgery.

CHAPTER 5

RECONSTRUCTION AND ALTERNATIVES

When you hear the word *reconstruction* you probably think "uh oh, implants." But because of the "Dow Disaster" and the billions of dollars Dow lost due to civil suits over its implant products, the entire breast reconstruction industry has changed. New technologies and surgical skills have resulted in some ingenious reconstruction techniques that don't use implants at all. Furthermore, not only are there safer implant products, such as saline, but new materials and implant products must meet much more stringent requirements before they gain market approval.

The purpose of this chapter is to cover all the various reconstructive techniques available, provide guidelines to finding a good surgeon and making the reconstruction decision, as well as to discuss some of the knowns and unknowns about the silicone implant, should you choose it. I will also outline alternatives to reconstructive surgery such as prostheses or just "going braless" (though this is not for everyone). I will even tell you where to get a "mastectomy-styled" bathing suit, thanks to an innovative Canadian designer.

But before I can cover what's new in reconstructive surgery, it is important to give you the background on the implant story. As you know, there are many credible critics of the implant lawsuits who maintain that the latest studies do not show any evidence of health problems linked to implant leakage or rupture. Nevertheless, until the complaints over silicone implants are absolutely disproved, you may not want to go near one. And of course, the idea of silicone oozing into your chest wall due to leakage or rupture is still disturbing—even if it doesn't cause connective tissue disease!

RECONSTRUCTION AND THE CIVIL WAR

It is estimated that roughly two million women in the United States alone have had implants; Canada and Europe account for several hundred thousand more. Eighty percent of all breast implant surgery is performed for cosmetic reasons (on women who want larger breasts); 20 percent is performed for reconstructive purposes on women who have had breast cancer surgery. But, technically, surgical alterations of breasts are always a reconstructive process. And as recently as 1981, the American Society of Plastic and Reconstructive Surgeons Inc. listed small breasts as a "disease."

Before silicone was invented, women injected paraffin, vegetable oil, lanolin, and even beeswax into their breasts to enlarge them. Surgeons began experimenting with glass balls in the 1930s and a variety of plastics in the 1950s. But the discovery of silicone for breast augmentation has an unlikely origin: Occupied Japan.

Japanese prostitutes who wanted a jump on their competition allowed themselves to be injected with industrial-strength, liquid silicone, which was designed for military use. The motivation was profit: American men were complaining about the small size of their breasts, so the bigger the breasts, the more business, they felt. This early experiment with silicone was disastrous. The silicone oozed out of the breasts and spread into the surrounding tissues. Years later, Japanese physicians described a new chronic fatigue-like condition called "human adjuvant disease"—a vague umbrella term that included a variety of the disorders we now call "connective tissue disease." This same disease is alleged to have a link to breast implants, which has caused most of the lawsuits. (This is discussed in detail on pages 160–163.)

When word got out about the new uses of silicone, manufacturing companies began experimenting with a variety of materials, methods, and chemicals for breast augmentation. One method involved using certain chemicals with silicone for the express purpose of forming scar tissue that would "hold in" the silicone. By the 1960s, thousands of women in North America and Europe were injected directly with silicone.

SILICONE VALLEY

Originally, all recipients of the silicone injections given in the 1960s were women who wanted larger breasts; a large group included wannabe showgirls and actresses. By the early 1960s, Dow Corning Corporation, the world's largest silicone supplier, set up a medical research center to further study the medical uses of silicone. In 1963, the Food and Drug Administration (FDA) gave Dow Corning the approval to do studies on liquid silicone in both animals and humans. The silicone-gel implant was introduced in 1965; it would eventually replace all direct silicone injections.

In 1967, it was reported that liquid silicone injections in monkeys and apes had caused massive damage to breast and surrounding tissues. Women who had been injected began to complain about lumps, rock-hard breasts, and silicone cysts. As a result, the FDA actually cancelled Dow Corning's research for two years, then consented again with the provision that Dow Corning could not inject silicone directly into women's breasts. By 1970, the FDA was authorized to regulate medical devices; but breast implants, through a technicality, were not on the list of medical devices because they were already on the market. In Canada, breast implants fell under "therapeutics" in the Food and Drug Act, which stipulated that a therapeutic had to be proved harmful before it could be banned.

Meme and the cancer alert

The first silicone implant to get bad press was the Meme. The Meme was not a Dow Corning product, but a product manufactured by New York City's Surgitek Inc., whose parent company was Bristol-Myers Squibb. Ironically, the product that preceded the Meme implant was designed by a surgeon named William J. Pangman, who was trying to find a way to rebuild breasts after cancer surgery. The Meme was a hot potato that kept being passed from one manufacturer to another. Surgitek bought Meme from Cooper Surgical, which had bought it from Natural-Y Surgical Specialities. Cooper had unloaded the Meme on Surgitek because studies showed that its polyurethane foam covering was releasing a cancer-causing compound, 2-4 toluene diamine (TDA), classified as "hazardous waste" by the U.S. Environmental Protection Agency (EPA).

Surgitek had other problems as well. In an FDA inspection that lasted sixteen days, it was discovered that Surgitek's implants, among other things, were not even sterile. It took eight months after the inspection for Surgitek to be ordered to clean up its act. Meme had still not been banned, however. Incredibly, even though the Meme had a horrible reputation among most surgeons, it managed to find a small market for itself. By 1989, several reports came out about the dangers of polyurethane, while many plastic surgeons were reporting infection rates as high as 20 percent after Meme implants. Finally, in March 1991, a New York City jury awarded a sixty-four-year-old single woman $4.45 million in the first damage suit linking the Meme to breast cancer. The woman had the Meme implanted in 1983 to lift her sagging breasts. She suffered inflammation for several weeks and had the Meme removed, but some of the foam had become entangled with her breast tissue when the Meme had ruptured, causing silicone to travel as far as her uterus. Although Bristol-Myers Squibb kept insisting the implant was safe, it was banned in 1991.

If you are one of the 200,000 women walking around with polyurethane foam-coated implants, you can have your urine tested for the carcinogen TDA. You must not breastfeed if you have this type of implant. The best thing to do is to have it replaced.

THE DOW INDUSTRIAL AVERAGES

The Meme ban in 1991 led many to question the safety of silicone implants. Every day, more women came forward with complaints of chronic joint pains, fatigue, rheumatoid arthritis-like symptoms, and a host of other ailments that doctors were calling "connective tissue disease" and "autoimmune disease."

These complaints, coupled with pending lawsuits over silicone leakage, caused FDA commissioner Dr. David Kessler to impose a temporary ban on silicone breast implants in January 1992. The ban was to stay in effect until more information on the safety of silicone implants was available on questions such as: How often did implants leak or rupture? Where does the silicone "travel" to in the body when it leaks? What happens to the body when it leaks? What are the long-term risks associated with leaks? News stories alleging that Dow Corning had neglected to carefully test its implant prior to marketing it started appearing. The reports quoted internal memos of Dow Corning which suggested that the company had implanted silicone in women before it had completed its animal studies, which were not even well-designed. The reports alleged that Dow's sales force had misled plastic surgeons over the safety of the implant. Two weeks after silicone implants were banned, Dow Corning announced that it would discontinue manufacturing breast implants. The cost of settling the various civil suits launched against Dow Corning had greatly affected its stock shares.

On February 10, 1992, Dow Corning released hundreds of internal documents that clearly showed a long history of health complaints over their implants. One memo in 1980 discussed a doctor's complaint about a "batch" of implants that were all leaking. In an effort to salvage its reputation, Dow Corning announced in March 1992 that it was not only getting out of the implant business altogether, but that it was releasing a series of compensation packages to women. In addition to setting up a $10 million fund to monitor breast implants in North American women who had received them, it would pay up to $1,200 to American women who could not afford surgical removal of the implants. Dow had only about $250 million in liability insurance, but there were reports that the company was facing more than $1 billion in lawsuits from American women.

In December 1993, a jury awarded Mariann Hopkins, forty-eight, $7.34 million in damages for breast implants she had had done in 1977 that had ruptured. Including this landmark suit, 9,000 individual lawsuits and 41 class action suits had been filed against Dow Corning Corporation and other implant manufacturers.

Call 1-800-PANIC

Lawyers began to circle in for the kill when they realized how lucrative the implant lawsuits were. Many firms advertised 1-800 numbers to get clients and organized large class action suits against the implant manufacturers. The ban and the lawsuits made some women so panicky that they actually attempted to cut out the implants themselves with razor blades if they couldn't afford explantation (removal of implants) by a qualified surgeon.

Law firms began to specialize in implant litigation. They accumulated miles of files of implant victims and had rooms filled with old implants in preservation fluids. One law firm even marketed workbooks and CD-ROM software as training tools to other law firms who wanted to learn how to litigate implant cases.

Soon, numerous "junk science" labs were marketing lab tests that could detect silicone in the bloodstream. Detecsil was a popular test that a surgeon proved was fraudulent. The surgeon sent blood from patients who did not wear implants, and found that no matter the age, sex, or implant history of a woman, Detecsil always came out positive! Unfortunately, these tests were submitted to a variety of United States courts as evidence of silicone contamination, and juries fell (and are still falling) for the results.

In addition, lawyers had no problem paying expert witnesses to back up claims that silicone was absolutely causing connective tissue and autoimmune disease in implant-wearers—even though this hadn't yet been proven by scientific studies and research.

The big three

In March 1994, Dow Corning, Bristol-Myers Squibb, and Baxter Healthcare announced the formation of the National Breast Implant Plaintiffs' Coalition, a joint compensation package. This global settlement package would provide more than $4 billion to women who had suffered ill health as a result of silicone breast implants. This fund would be distributed over a thirty-year period, and would cover roughly 80 percent of the estimated $4 billion settlement costs. Breast implant recipients could either reject or accept the offer; they could pursue their insurance claims if they did not like the offer. The payments depended on age and the severity of medical problems. The younger the claimant, the more money would be paid over her lifetime.

1995: THE YEAR OF THE SCIENCE

Between 1993 and 1995, reports questioning whether connective tissue disease was indeed linked to breast implants began to trickle into medical journals. The results were coming in negative—even though some epidemiologists were hoping for other results. Just before the deadline for women to sign up for the global settlement package, the Mayo Clinic published the largest study of its time on the link between connective tissue disease and silicone. It found no link.

This infuriated implant-wearers and lawyers, who insisted that the study was rigged and had been bought and paid for by pharmaceutical companies. The medical community insisted that receiving educational grants from pharmaceutical companies was commonplace, and there were always rigid rules in place that stipulated that the arrangement had no strings attached.

By 1995, studies from all over the world, including a very credible Harvard University study, were showing results consistent with the Mayo Clinic study. Ironically, the more the scientific community said there was no link to connective tissue disease, the more lawsuits implant manufacturers were losing.

Lawyers allege that the studies are based on "traditional" criteria for classic autoimmune or connective tissue disease. They argue that since implants seem to be causing a new host of symptoms that are related but not limited to connective tissue disease, perhaps there is a brand new disease studies should be looking into. The medical community rejects this argument, however. A wild hypothesis, which showed up in a 1997 edition of the *Journal of the American Medical Association,* suggests that hair dye and NOT breast implants may be the culprit behind connective tissue disease, because (get this), hair dyes are not only also linked to these symptoms, but women with implants are more likely to use hair dye.

SILICONE AND BREAST CANCER

Breast cancer patients were *not* happy about the implant ban at all. They felt that the ban denied them their right to rebuild not just their bodies, but their lives. In North America, the ban has been lifted only for experimental research and for women needing breast reconstruction after breast cancer surgery—so long as they are followed closely after implant surgery. It is thought that the therapeutic benefits of "wholeness" outweigh the still unproven health risks associated with silicone rupture. The lifting of the ban also extends to women who require reconstruction after accidents or due to physical deformities (congenital or otherwise).

Roughly 20 percent of all reconstructive surgery is performed to replace a breast lost to cancer surgery. Fortunately, as a result of the implant controversy, other methods of reconstruction are being made available.

IMPLANT-FREE RECONSTRUCTION

Reconstruction is usually best performed at the time of an initial mastectomy. Your specialists and plastic surgeon should discuss your treatment and reconstruction options with you. You can have any of these procedures done at any time after cancer surgery. Some women decide to have the surgery as late as two decades after their initial mastectomy. And that's just fine. In any event, discuss your preferences regarding the timing of your reconstruction with your surgeon, who will be able to guide you accordingly.

Since the implant controversy is still unsettled, and hence is still unsettling for many women, I'll cover all the non-implant techniques first, then list all the implants currently on the market. It is worth noting that not all women can have implants put in, even though they want them. This is because there often isn't enough breast tissue left after a mastectomy to enable a surgeon to work with the implant. If too much skin and muscle is removed in the cancer surgery, the skin may not be elastic enough to allow for an implant. In addition, radiation therapy (see Chapter 4) can dramatically affect the area's elasticity, too. Sometimes a tissue expansion procedure is done to get around this (see page 173).

And finally, if you want the breast to have a rebuilt nipple and areola, additional procedures may be done that combine both non-implant and implant surgery.

All implant-free reconstruction involves a surgery known as myocutaneous flaps: *myo* literally means muscle, while *cutaneous* means skin. This procedure involves moving tissue from one part of the body to the site of the mastectomy. It also entails two incisions, major surgery, and a longer recovery time. While these procedures are more complex than traditional implant procedures, they don't involve placing anything foreign into your body that has unproven risk factors. Using real tissue also makes for softer, more real-feeling breasts in the end.

Finally, the recent cloning of Dolly the sheep may yield some exciting possibilities for breast reconstruction. Right now, research is underway to "clone" a breast using a woman's own cells to grow new breast tissue. This is years away from perfection, but surely, a breast is easier to clone than a whole sheep!

THE ABDOMINIZER: THE TRAM FLAP

One of the more ingenious procedures invented is the abdominal flap or TRAM flap, shown in figure 5.1. Here, you pay for a breast reconstruction procedure but get a free tummy tuck thrown in (although a true tummy tuck would not leave as much of a scar or discomfort). (This procedure was shown on The Learning Channel's "The Operation" and is available on video if you call.)

Under a general anesthetic, a new breast is created with your own "ab flab." TRAM stands for transverse rectus abdominus muscle. Transverse refers to the surgical cut, which is horizontal as opposed to vertical; rectus abdominus muscle is the stuff of which tummy flab is made. Here's what's involved:

1. The surgeon makes a "bikini cut" across your abdomen (hip-to-hip, similar to what's done in a cesarean section, but more extensive).
2. The surgeon makes an incision at the mastectomy scar line, which acts as a flap.
3. The surgeon sews the fatty abdominal tissue, along with a supplying blood vessel, into the blood vessel in the axilla (armpit).

Figure 5.1

TYPES OF IMPLANT-FREE RECONSTRUCTION PROCEDURES

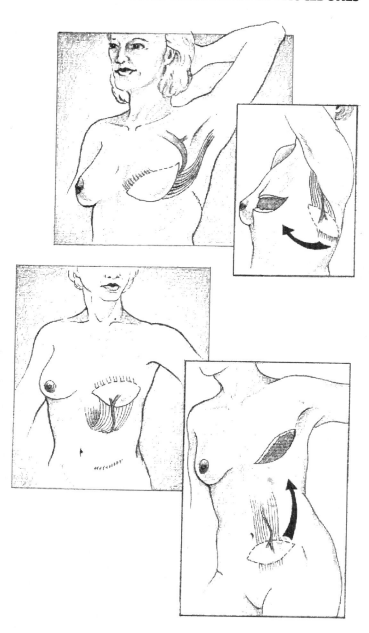

4. The surgeon "stuffs" the chest incision with your tummy "stuffing."

5. The surgeon uses the abdominal skin left over to cover the new breast mound. (Nipple reconstruction is discussed later.)

The procedure takes three to six hours to do; the hospital stay averages about five to seven days.

The aftereffects

Well, you will have a new breast that is more or less a good match to your existing breast. However, because this is major surgery, it has all the complications that go with major surgery: anesthetic risks, fatigue, etc. And because this procedure is more extensive than a basic implant, there is a longer recovery period.

The tummy tuck will certainly leave you with less abdominal flab—a bonus, if you will—but it can weaken the abdominal wall, which can weaken abdominal muscle strength and lead to a serious condition, such as a hernia. These days, most surgeons will replace the muscle they remove with fake muscle made out of a plastic material. If this isn't offered, ask for it. Blood clots and lung problems after surgery are also possible.

Who isn't a TRAM candidate?

Thin women. If you have a completely flat and toned abdomen, there simply won't be enough fat and loose muscle to work with. At one time, the TRAM was not done on women who had had previous abdominal surgery such as a cesarean section. But this is changing. You will need to check with your surgeon if previous abdominal surgery is a contraindication. If you are too thin to have a TRAM, you may be able to have the latissimus dorsi flap procedure (tissue from the back), which is discussed in the next section.

In addition, any woman who is not physically well enough to weather major surgery cannot have the TRAM. Your health status will depend on how much adjuvant therapy you have had and how well you have responded. And because of the risk of blood clots and lung problems after surgery, smokers and diabetics are not good candidates, either.

Variations on the theme

In some cases, the surgeon can use the skin and fat from the midriff, the area just below the breast, and leave the abdominal area intact. This will leave a more visible scar, so you won't look perfect in a bikini, but this type of flap surgery avoids using any muscle, and the skin color may be a better match, too.

Other variations involve improving the symmetry of the breasts. This may mean additional procedures on the rebuilt breast; in the case of very large-breasted women, it could mean doing a breast reduction procedure on the other breast. In this case, breast tissue from the other breast could also be used to rebuild the missing breast.

The TRAM can also be used to create a pocket for an implant in cases where there is not enough breast tissue left to support an implant.

What to expect

Reconstruction surgery can create a close match of the other breast, but the new breast is rarely an exact match. (If you've had a double mastectomy, asymmetry will not be as much of a problem in reconstruction.) A woman with one natural breast and one rebuilt breast may have a difficult time getting used to the rebuilt breast, especially since there is no feeling in the rebuilt breast. A breast rebuilt with the TRAM procedure will feel more like a real breast to the touch than a breast with an implant, although it will still take some getting used to.

BACK TO FRONT: LATISSIMUS DORSI FLAP

Shown in figure 5.2, this is an older version of the TRAM flap procedure in which skin, muscle, fat, and the blood vessels that nourish them are taken from the back instead of the abdominal area and literally moved around to the chest area. The procedure got its name from the latissimus dorsi muscle, of which the lower back is made. The procedure was originally invented as a way to build tissue into the chest that could hold an implant, but it can also be used to reconstruct the breast without an implant, so long as there's enough fat to work with from the back. Here's what's involved:

Figure 5.2
TRAM FLAP AND LATISSIMUS DORSI FLAP PROCEDURES

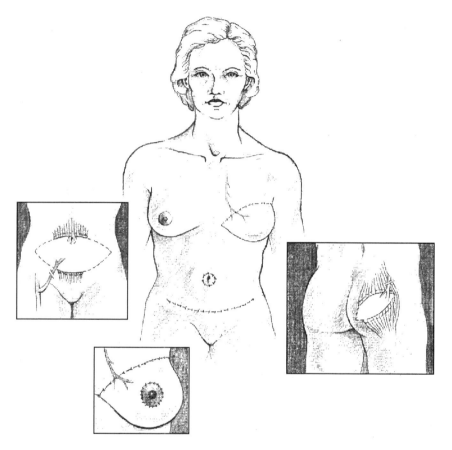

1. The surgeon makes an incision in your back, which eventually becomes a long, thin scarline.
2. The surgeon moves the back tissue around to the chest area and builds a pocket out of it at the mastectomy site.
3. The surgeon "stuffs" the pocket with the back tissue. (An implant can also be inserted in the pocket.)

The procedure takes as much time as the TRAM flap—three to six hours. The hospital stay is about the same as well, five to seven days.

The aftereffects

Recuperation time for the latissimus dorsi flap procedure is roughly six weeks. All the major risks associated with the TRAM flap surgery are present in this procedure as well. There is a chance that the blood vessels feeding the flap could block up, in which case the tissue used for the procedure would die and the flap will not hold in place properly. This surgery also results in loss of the latissimus muscle in the lower back, but many women don't notice this change as much as they notice weakness in the shoulders, which causes them to droop.

Who should not have this done?

As with the TRAM flap, women who cannot handle the strain of major surgery are not good candidates for this procedure. Women who suffer from chronic back pain or a back problem should find out whether this procedure will aggravate their problem before they have surgery.

A NEW NIPPLE

Nipple reconstruction is usually done after a flap procedure, but it can be done simultaneously as well. Some women don't bother with this procedure at all and are satisfied with a rebuilt breast mound.

Building materials

To make a new nipple, a surgeon can use skin and connective tissue from the inner thigh, chest, groin, or earlobe. Sometimes a nipple can be constructed with existing nipple tissue from the other breast. After the nipple is built, a special tattooing procedure can be done that dyes the area surrounding the nipple so that it look like an authentic areola. This procedure can be done in the surgeon's office.

How does the new breast feel?

You will not have any feeling in the breast, but to a lover, it will feel soft and natural, just like a real breast, because it's made with your own tissue. And, with a reconstructed breast, there is no need to worry about rupture or leakage. If you've had all your breast tissue removed, your new breast should remain unchanged throughout your cycle and even during pregnancy (if you're still menstruating). If you do have some breast tissue left, the tissue may respond to the hormonal changes in your body and enlarge during periods and pregnancies. This may temporarily affect symmetry with the other breast. Or, the asymmetry could be caused by your remaining breast, which may stay enlarged throughout a cycle.

A CONSUMER'S GUIDE TO BREAST IMPLANTS

Implant procedures involve far less surgery than non-implant procedures. An implant procedure involves making a small incision at the site of the mastectomy, into which the implant is inserted and sewn into place. Most women today opt for saline (salt water) implants because these don't appear to have any of the risks involved with leakage or rupture—saline implants can rupture, but all that leaks out is salt water, which is not dangerous to your health in any way. There are other types of implants in addition to saline, and a few different techniques to insert them. One of the newer methods involves tissue expansion, which is done when there isn't enough tissue left to work with. Tissue expansion is discussed in detail further on.

HAVING YOUR FILL

In the same way that all tires are made out of rubber, all implants are encased in a rubber-like material called elastomer, rubberized silicone; the polyurethane foam encasing has been permanently banned. But it is not the shell of the implant that determines the implant's performance but its filling. Some fillings are more apt to leak or rupture than others, and a few fillings, like silicone, are considered to be toxic to the body when they leak. So when you are shopping for implants, make sure it is the fillings you look at. There are basically three varieties of implants:

- *Silicone gel.* Silicone is a synthetic plastic that can take the form of a liquid (discussed at the beginning of this chapter), a gel, or an elastomer. The gel is clear and jelly-like in consistency, which makes it a good material to create a lifelike breast from. Prior to the ban on silicone use in the general population (with the noted exceptions of breast cancer patients, and patients with breast deformities), it was pretty much the only implant used (silicone is also available in a variety of sizes). Today, the risks of illnesses linked to rupture or leakage are making silicone candidates wary. The risks of silicone are discussed separately on page 174.

- *Saline.* As mentioned earlier, saline is just sterile salt water. An empty envelope is implanted first. The surgeon then adds the salt water. The saline is added after the implant is put into place because this makes for easier sizing and surgery. Saline is certainly a safer option than silicone, but its track record suggests that it is a weak second in terms of consistency and natural appearance. Saline wearers complain that the breast doesn't hang or look as natural as a silicone breast and that the implant can look "wrinkly" under the skin. Deflation is another problem. Over time, saline can leak out (which *isn't* dangerous), affecting the shape of the implant, which could require replacement surgery. However, there are plenty of surgeons and patients who swear by saline implants and feel that its safety is worth the small sacrifices. The insertion scar is also smaller with a saline implant because the implant envelope is put in deflated.

- *Double lumen implants.* Lumen refers to the outer envelope that holds in the filling. This is the "double bagger" silicone gel implant. The implant is encased in an elastomer envelope, which is again encased in an elastomer envelope in case there is a leak or a rupture. In some styles, the inner envelope is prefilled with silicone gel, while the outer envelope is filled with saline during implantation. Or you can have the reverse: saline on the inside; silicone on the outside. Some surgeons think this version is less likely to cause capsular contracture, discussed later.

THE IMPLANT PROCEDURE

Surgery for implant insertion is not very complicated. It involves one simple incision around the site of the mastectomy, after which the implant is inserted behind or underneath the pectoralis major muscle (a.k.a. chest muscle). Women who have this procedure for augmentation have the implant inserted between the breast and the chest muscle.

The incision's location varies from woman to woman, depending on the kind of mastectomy she has had (see Chapter 4), her general body shape, and her own preference. For example, in an augmentation procedure, the incision is often hidden under the crease of the breast. In reconstruction, the surgeon simply follows the scarline of the mastectomy.

And unlike the non-implant procedures discussed earlier, this is a much simpler surgery that can even be done under a local anesthetic. When it is done under a general anesthetic, it's done as day surgery (you can go home the same day). If you're having a bad reaction to the anesthetic, or you've developed an infection around your scarline, you may need to stay overnight in the hospital, however.

What to expect after implant surgery

A surgical bra or bandage will be placed over your incision for about ten days. During this healing period, you may experience some swelling, a little pain, or discomfort. Analgesics such as acetaminophen should take care of these symptoms. During this time, you should also avoid strenuous activities that would place a strain on your chest muscles. So lifting heavy weights and push-ups are not recommended!

The implant breast will be rounder, higher, and firmer than your natural breast, but it may also be a little smaller—it all depends on how much tissue your surgeon had to work with. If you're not happy with the match, you can sometimes have reduction surgery on the opposite breast, or if it's a case of sagging, you can have what's called "uplift" surgery.

TISSUE EXPANSION

Have you ever had a pair of leather shoes stretched? Well, tissue expansion works on the same principle. Sometimes it is just not possible to have a simple implant procedure because there isn't enough tissue to work with, which is the case if you've had a modified radical mastectomy. So your surgeon will suggest you have a tissue expansion procedure prior to the implant surgery.

Tissue expansion is done by making an incision at the mastectomy scar to create a pocket and then inserting the empty elastomer shell of a saline implant. Saline will be added very gradually over a period of about eight to twelve weeks. The saline is injected into the implant's shell through a special tube, which causes the shell to expand and inflate over a longer course of time. The expander has a special filling device that will be removed under a local anesthetic once your breast has inflated to the size you need. After the filling device is removed, an internal valve that's built into the implant shuts automatically, creating a normal-sized, permanent implant.

The size of inflation you want may not always be possible, however, so many times the result is a smaller breast than you'd like.

THE TROUBLE WITH IMPLANTS

While many women experience no problems with their implants, clearly there are many who do. Close to half a million women in the United States report illnesses that they link to breast implants. In addition, roughly 25 percent of all women with breast implants will develop local complications that may require more surgery. The complications are higher in women who had implants for reconstructive reasons. These complications range from implant "sweating" or leaking, rupture, or problems with the site of surgery, such as bleeding, infection, and so on. Surgeons also report more complications with reconstruction surgery after a mastectomy because of the initial trauma to the area: tighter skin, less tissue, and so on. So what exactly are the problems with breast implants? Here's a list in alphabetical order.

Calcium deposits

Regardless of whether you have silicone or saline, calcium can form in the tissue surrounding the implant. Pain and breast hardening is the end result, but your health is not in endangered.

Capsular contracture

Depending on what you read, anywhere from 10 to 70 percent of women experience capsular contracture within about six months of implant surgery—be it silicone or saline. A capsular contraction occurs when the scar tissue formed around the implant as a reaction to the foreign matter inside forms a tight capsule that squeezes the implant and makes the breast feel very hard and uncomfortable. This makes it difficult to do things like sleeping on your front or even hugging. This can lead to pain and a deformed-looking breast. As miserable as this is, your overall health is not in danger from capsular contracture.

Connective Tissue Disease

This is an umbrella term that is being used to describe a variety of health problems that are believed to be linked to silicone. See the separate section on page 176.

Leaking and rupture

As discussed throughout this chapter, yes, all implants can leak or rupture with age. This is why the FDA has banned silicone gel implants for the general public (see earlier pages in this chapter), and this is why saline was even developed as an implant filler. The difference between silicone gel and saline is that since saline is just sterile salt water, if it leaks out or ruptures, no harm is done (you will need to have the implant replaced, however). But if silicone gel leaks out or ruptures, there is a risk that you may experience dire health problems, thrown under the umbrella term *connective tissue disease*. This is discussed further on.

What causes leaking or rupture? Trauma to the breast (such as the kind of pressure exerted during a mammogram) is cited as one cause, but most experts believe that leaking and rupture are linked to wear and tear—in other words, the age of your implant. Given this fact, you may want to replace your implant every ten years or so, as pacemakers are.

For the moment, there are no clear answers about how often and why implants leak or rupture, but we do know that implants made between 1975 and 1986 have a much worse track record because their outer shells were made of a thinner material and the silicone gel has more liquid. Nor are there clear statistics about how many women have experienced leaks or ruptures, although some data points to significant percentages.

Another problem with ruptures and leaks is that you may not notice it's happened. Generally, the more scar tissue that forms around your implant, the more contained your leak or rupture will be. This may be why only some women with ruptures suffer from health problems.

Worse is a phenomenon known as "gel bleed," which is a fact of life with silicone implants. Gel bleed is the seeping of silicone through the outer shell in such small quantities that the word *leak* isn't really accurate. But gel bleed can be tantamount to getting daily injections of silicone in microscopic amounts, which would explain why some women can experience health problems even when no rupture or leak is detected. See the separate section on detecting leaks on page 178.

Obvious signs of leakage or rupture include small lumps in the breast or chest area, known as granulomas, or swollen lymph nodes under the arms (caused by loose silicone that the body is trying to fight). Also watch for tenderness or discomfort around the implant and a change in the shape, movement, or consistency of the breast. Call your surgeon if you suspect a rupture. Experts advise that the next step is getting the implant removed and having the area around the implant rupture cleaned out.

Mammography complications

When you have a silicone or saline implant, it is harder to get an accurate mammogram because cancerous lumps can be hidden by the implants. And if you have scar tissue or calcium deposits around the implant, this may interfere with the interpretation of the mammogram. See Chapter 2 for more information on maximizing mammography.

ABOUT CONNECTIVE TISSUE DISEASE

Sometimes referred to as autoimmune disease (meaning that the body attacks itself), connective tissue disease describes a variety of aches and pains that many experts link to silicone implant rupture or leakage. (Again, studies to date do not show a link.) The symptoms can take the form of rheumatoid arthritis-like joint pain, lupus-like inflammation, rashes, or flu-like symptoms and fatigue that are similar to the symptoms of chronic fatigue syndrome. The problem with connective tissue disease is that for every credible expert that believes it is linked to silicone, there is another equally credible expert who refutes the charge.

In addition, some experts are linking a host of autoimmune diseases such as scleroderma, rheumatoid arthritis, lupus, and chronic fatigue syndrome directly to implants. In other words, it is believed that the silicone in the implants is somehow triggering off these diseases because it is creating an "autoimmune war" within the body. Some experts believe that women who are genetically predisposed to autoimmune diseases increase their risk of developing the disease when silicone leaks or ruptures. This is yet to be proven, however, and many experts feel that there is simply no credible data that can make the claim in spite of a 1997 Tulane study that discovered an anti-polymer antibody present in women with autoimmune disease symptoms.

Given what we know about the immune system's reaction to foreign tissue in the body (such as the formation of scar tissue around an implant), and given the fact that silicone can travel throughout the body after a rupture or leak, the idea that you might not feel well after a silicone implant rupture isn't as outlandish as critics make it sound. Furthermore, animal studies have shown that silicone gel may cause inflammatory reactions in the body; in Japan, women exhibited the same symptoms of connective tissue disease two decades before the lawsuits against implant manufacturers were launched.

How many women are affected?

The data surrounding connective tissue disease is not clear. It appears as though the number of women with the symptoms of connective tissue disease is the same in both implant and non-implant wearers. But opponents of silicone implants believe that the symptoms of connective tissue disease are so vague, and take so long to develop, that it is too early to tell.

Proving or disproving the link

There are a number of problems with making the link between silicone and connective tissue disease. First, since autoimmune disorders have a habit of improving on their own, it is not easy to isolate why patients seem to feel better when implants are removed.

Scientifically, silicone is considered to be biologically inert, meaning that, in theory, it shouldn't be harmful when it comes into contact with human tissue. And this has been proven by the use of silicone in other areas of medicine: as a lubricant in hypodermic needles, as a coating for pacemakers, as the main ingredient in artificial joints, and in over-the-counter medicines and baby formula (although formula-fed infants generally have many more health problems than breastfed infants).

While most experts agree that there is no link between silicone and breast cancer, there is continuing disagreement over the link between connective tissue disease and silicone. As discussed on page 163, several studies since 1993, including the Harvard University and the Mayo Clinic studies, were not able to establish a link between connective tissue disease and silicone—and these were considered to be good studies.

What should you do?

Until we know more about silicone and connective tissue disease, it is best to stay alert to the possible signs and symptoms. The main symptoms to watch for are the kind of symptoms that you should report to your doctor anyway, given your cancer diagnosis; many of these symptoms can also mask the side effects of other therapies. They include: muscle and joint pain, which could be a sign of inflammation; skin changes such as tightness, redness, rashes, thickening, hardening, or swelling (particularly around the breasts); swollen glands or lymph nodes (swollen nodes can also indicate a recurrence); unusual, extreme, or unexplained fatigue (which may also be related to your chemotherapy or surgery); edema (swelling), particularly in your hands and feet; and hair loss (which could be related to your chemotherapy).

Which doctor do you contact if you suspect a leak or rupture?

The surgeon who performed your reconstructive surgery is the first doctor you should·contact. You may also wish to consult with a rheumatologist or your medical oncologist (to rule out symptoms that may be drug reactions). An allergist may also be a good contact down the road. A consumer group called the Command Trust Network (see the appendix) can suggest appropriate specialists for your symptoms as well as send you good literature.

FINDING A LEAK

If you have a saline implant, the breast will usually deflate when the implant breaks (one of the problems with saline, as outlined earlier). But with silicone gel, the breasts don't always deflate with a leak or rupture. That's why it is important to have regular follow-up exams with your surgeon, gynecologist, internist, or any doctor who performs manual breast exams. All these practitioners are trained to look for subtle changes that may indicate a leak or rupture.

Unfortunately, mammograms are not good detection tools and are useless at finding leaks or ruptures. CAT scans or MRIs are also not reliable at picking up leaks or ruptures. Manual exams are your best bet.

Apparently, some hospitals find that ultrasound is a good tool to confirm or rule out a rupture or leak. Ultrasound can also be used to detect silicone in the axillary (armpit) lymph nodes, but it is not recommended as a screening method. In addition, significant training is required to read sonograms to distinguish the unique pattern indicating a silicone leak.

Things to keep in mind

It is important to be frank about your implant in certain circumstances. For example, anytime you have a mammogram, you need to let the technicians know that you wear an implant. That's because you will need to have less compression on your breast to avoid rupture; the breast will need to be X rayed from more angles for accuracy; and you will need to have the mammogram read by a radiologist who is trained in reading implants. Any facility that's been certified by the American College of Radiology should be fine.

And, of course, it is important to let the doctor who is performing a manual breast exam know that you have implants (if it is not obvious).

ALTERNATIVES TO RECONSTRUCTION

Since there are considerable drawbacks to reconstructive surgery, you may just want to forget it and opt for an alternative: a breast prosthesis (a replacement breast worn under clothing) or wearing nothing. This decision is highly subjective and depends on the kind of mastectomy you've had (radical or modified; single or double) as well as the size of the remaining breast. But your body image, personal preference, and lifestyle will have more to do with your decision.

HOW TO FIND A GOOD PROSTHESIS

If you want to appear as if you have two breasts but don't want to go through breast reconstruction, a breast prosthesis is a great option.

You will probably get a temporary prosthesis while you're still in the hospital. However this is not a high-quality product but a "filler" until you make your decision. (These temps are donated by the Reach to Recovery program, which, for the most part, doesn't have the best track record when it comes to real patient support.) These interim prostheses are made out of a fluffy material that can adjust to your shape and size. They look fine under clothing, but there are much higher quality prostheses out there that will look more realistic.

Where to shop

You probably won't find breast prostheses or mastectomy bras at Victoria's Secret, but more department stores and specialty lingerie shops are stocking items for mastectomy survivors. (Often the owners of small shops have had mastectomies themselves.) To save some time, let your fingers do the walking first. Check your yellow pages for these buzzwords: *Brassieres, Prostheses, Surgical Supplies or Appliances,* or even *Mastectomy Products.* You can also look under *Specialty Lingerie* or *Specialty Undergarments.* Specialty medical supply "yellow pages" have also been put out by various companies that have

Figure 5.3

WHAT A BREAST FORM MIGHT LOOK LIKE INSIDE YOUR BRA

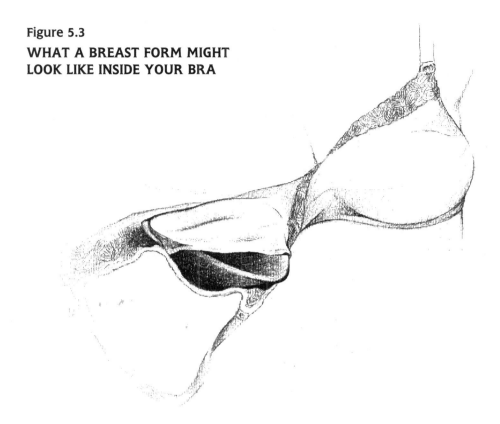

exhaustive listings of all kinds of medical supply manufacturers and retailers. The best one is Medi-Pages; you can get it by calling 1-800-554-6661. Local support groups and non-profit organizations can also tell you where to shop for prostheses and mastectomy bras in your area. Some organizations have samples they can show you and even provide regular demonstrations and seminars on prostheses so you know what to look for and what to expect when you make your purchase. And, of course, your breast surgeon can recommend a few places, too.

Silicone... again!

For the same reasons that silicone makes the best-looking implants, it also makes the best-looking prosthesis. It also feels like a natural breast. All prostheses come in a variety of sizes and shapes to match your existing breast. They can also vary in weight firmness and can fit either side (right or left).

You can also find prostheses to fill in the gaps left by any of the mastectomy procedures discussed in Chapter 3. Some are designed to replace breasts, while others can fill in gaps made by partial mastectomies. If you've had a partial mastectomy, you're probably looking for a silicone shell with a built-in nipple. You can also use partial prostheses to fill in gaps from implant surgery or reconstruction. As for nipples, some prostheses have built-in nipples while others require a separate purchase. You'll find the nipple at the same place that sells the prosthesis and mastectomy bras.

You can find a high-quality prosthesis for roughly U.S. $200 to $300. And yes, you *can* get a prescription for a prosthesis, which means that your insurance can cover at least some of the cost. Many breast cancer organizations now have funds available for women who can't afford a prosthesis. See the appendix for listings of such organizations.

Custom-made prostheses are also available. You'll need to call around to various prostheses stores to find out where you can get one; your surgeon and breast cancer support organizations are also good sources of information. Getting a prosthesis custom-made is similar to getting dentures. A mold of your chest is made so the prosthesis can fit the shape of your body and match your other breast exactly. The drawbacks are time and money. You need to go back several times for fittings; the cost is roughly U.S. $2,000.

Tips for shoppers

When you're shopping around for a prosthesis, it is best to comparison shop. In other words, don't buy the first one you try on; there may be other styles that are more comfortable.

A good prosthesis should not only feel comfortable, but it should stay put when you move, stretch, reach, and so on. Interestingly, experts recommend wearing a tight-fitting sweater or spandex-like top when you shop so you know exactly what the prosthesis will look like in the "toughest" clothing. This will also give you a chance to compare how it looks against the other breast. You will also want to make sure that the prosthesis is level with the other breast and that the built-in nipple (if it has one) matches your natural nipple in "area circumference."

Finally, make sure you find out about any warranty that may come with the prosthesis in case you need to replace it.

Going braless

While most of you will want a mastectomy bra, there are adhesives you can buy that keep the prostheses in place. These adhesives also allow for more freedom in clothing styles—especially strapless clothing and bathing suits. In the past, only liquid adhesives, which needed to be applied daily, were available. But now you can get Velcro-inspired adhesives, one side sticks on your chest, the other on the prosthesis. These are called attachable breast forms. You'll find these adhesives at the same places that stock mastectomy bras and prostheses. These special tapes need to be replaced every week or so, but showering, sleeping, or swimming won't interfere with them.

The only side effect of an adhesive like this is a possible allergy to the tape. So always do a skin test first when you use an adhesive—and do it away from your mastectomy site. Radiation can also make your skin more sensitive to adhesives.

Designer bathing suits

There is now a special line of designer mastectomy-styled bathing suits made by award-winning Canadian designer Linda Lundstrom. (One of my own countrywomen!) The line is called "Survivor Swim Wear" and is available at the stores listed under "Swimwear" in the appendix at the back of the book or by calling 1-800-66-LINDA for more information.

All these one-piece bathing suits come with special inner pockets that adjust to various prosthesis sizes. Special stitching has been added to the bustline so you can adjust the size of the pocket that fits the prosthesis. What's interesting about this line is that it is identical to Lundstrom's regular line of swim wear. All come in vibrant colors, matching cover-robes, and other accessories. Lundstrom ties a tiny pink ribbon to the mastectomy-styled bathing suits so women can shop discreetly. The suits are both functional and fashionable.

WEARING NOTHING

Wearing nothing is a comfortable option for a growing segment of mastectomy survivors. However, if you're large-breasted, a lopsided chest could cause some strain to your back, shoulders, or neck. Some women wear a prosthesis just to alleviate the strain, but if you're comfortable with nothing, you may never need a prosthesis for this purpose. Here are some guidelines that may increase your psychological and physical comfort:

- Choose clothing that you're comfortable with. Whether it's looser tops or layers (blazers and sweaters), don't feel pressured to specifically hide your surgery by something you normally would not wear.
- If you're experiencing back, neck, or shoulder strain, consult a physical therapist. You may be able to do some exercises to relieve the strain if you don't want to wear a prosthesis.

MAKING AN INFORMED DECISION

It seems as though the experience of breast cancer is making one series of decisions after another. Not only do you have all the decisions about treatment and adjuvant therapy to make, but you are now faced with the complexities of replacing your breast.

If you're exploring the idea of having either a non-implant procedure (see page 164) or an implant procedure (see page 172), here are some guidelines that will help you make the right decision.

SHOPTALK

If you're considering the surgery route, you will need to talk to a surgeon before you make your final decision. So be sure to:

- Shop around for a surgeon. Your breast cancer surgeon may be qualified to do reconstruction, but often you need to find a plastic surgeon.

- Interview at least two plastic surgeons so you can get a feel for the difference in approaches that are out there.
- Double-check that your plastic surgeon is a board-certified plastic surgeon.
- Find out how many breast reconstructions your plastic surgeon has done in the past year and compare the numbers. Obviously, the more she's done, the better. Then find out how experienced the surgeon is in the particular procedure you want done.
- Ask to see your surgeon's "photo album" so you can see the before and after shots of women who've had the particular surgery you are considering. Look for pictures of women with similar body shapes to yours.
- Ask the surgeon for pictures of the worst case scenario, too.
- Get as much literature as you can on the kind of procedure and implant you are considering, and so on.
- Draw up a pros and con list about all the options: saline versus silicone; flap procedures versus implants; prosthesis versus implants; and so on.

IF YOU WANT IMPLANTS

It is worthwhile to find out if you have a family history of autoimmune disorders. That way, you'll be prepared for signs of the disorder in case the implant triggers it. Common autoimmune disorders that some experts believe can be triggered by implants are lupus, scleroderma, and rheumatoid arthritis.

You should avoid implants if you have a history of allergy or sensitivity to foreign materials.

It is also important to seek out other implant-wearers to gather quotes and listen to their experiences. If they had to do it over again, would they make the same decision?

ARE THE CUSTOMERS SATISFIED?

A number of studies have looked at the value of reconstructive surgery. For the most part, yes, the customers are satisfied. One study looked at the timing issue: Does immediate reconstruction offer any benefit over delaying the procedure?

Interestingly, there was no difference in terms of ultimate satisfaction, but the women who delayed reconstruction suffered more from depression and anxiety prior to the reconstruction.

Another study found that women who had reconstruction immediately were able to accept their appearance more easily than those who delayed reconstruction. (But this seems like a rather obvious result!)

A specific survey that looked at just implants found that 90 percent of the respondents felt that the implants had freed them from the inconvenience of a prosthesis; 80 percent felt that the implants made them whole again; 55 percent said implants helped make the breast cancer experience go away.

· · · · · · ·

Although reconstructive surgery is something you must contemplate on your own, too often it is undertaken only for the sexual partner. How do partners, spouses, and lovers cope with breast cancer, and what can they do to help you through the experience? And how exactly does breast cancer change your sex life? You'll find out in the next chapter.

CHAPTER 6

FRIENDS AND LOVERS

Breast cancer is a family disease—not in the sense that it is genetic (which it is), but in the sense that it affects the entire family and all your loved ones surrounding you. Many women going through breast cancer feel estranged from their loved ones, and vice versa. This is why breast cancer sometimes breaks marriages and relationships. But it doesn't have to. With the expertise of breast cancer survivors, spouses of breast cancer patients, psycho-oncologists (psychiatrists specializing in cancer patient therapy), and a range of breast cancer therapists, this chapter outlines key communication tools you can use with your significant other to work through the experience of breast cancer in as healthy a manner as possible. It also discusses valuable ways spouses and partners can help you. I encourage you to show your partner this chapter when you're finished with it, and use it as a tool to open up the lines of communication.

The latter half of this chapter also discusses sexual concerns. How does breast cancer change your sex life and fertility? What can you do to overcome the loss of your breast(s) in your sexual experience with your partner? A variety of these complex issues are discussed.

Since so much of our communication is through "subtexts," I've presented some of the information in this chapter a little differently from previous chapters.

THE SPOUSAL SCENE

FADE IN: Oncology waiting area. The mood is somber. The waiting area is packed. Men and women, alone and together, of all races and ages sit together, whispering quietly. Jane and John Doe are in their mid-forties. Jane has breast cancer. She has just finished a regimen of chemo and has lost her hair. She wears a silk scarf around her head. John holds her hand.

JANE: Who's going to pick up Tara?

JOHN: Your sister. She'll take her to ballet and then out for a bite.

JANE: My car needs an oil change.

JOHN: I'll take care of it.... You finding out the results of your blood tests today?

JANE: Uh huh.

JOHN: You had a good white count the last time, didn't you?

JANE: Uh huh.

[*Long pause*]

JOHN: God, It's always such a long wait! Even when we get here early.

JANE: It won't be much longer now.

[*Long pause*]

VOICE: Jane *Doe?*

JANE: [*Grabbing her purse*] That's me!

JOHN: [*Lets go of her hand*] I'll be waiting.

[*Jane leaves John sitting in the waiting area and heads into the examination rooms. John gets up and paces. Picks up an issue of* Time *and tosses it down in disgust. It's a year old.*]

    FADE OUT.

What you just read is a composite of the experiences spouses of breast cancer patients relay. I call it the spousal scene because it seems to be a universal experience of spouses or partners who love a woman with breast cancer.

In this scene, John and Jane are a model couple, braving the breast cancer experience, trying to carry on as normally as possible. Jane makes sure John has taken care of the small details in life: arranging her eight-year-old daughter's schedule, fixing the car. John, on the other hand, is trying to participate in Jane's therapy. He feebly attempts to find out as much as possible from Jane about her last appointment and what information will be revealed today. Jane doesn't want to talk about it. For one thing, Jane isn't feeling well enough to recall every single thing her medical oncologist tells her in these appointments. Jane doesn't like talking about this sort of thing in public, with thirty other people around. But what happens to John when Jane goes to her appointment and he's left behind in the waiting area? He feels more and more cut off from her experience, and more and more impotent as a spouse. Jane, alone in the oncology appointment room, becomes more and more overwhelmed by the experience and less able to talk about it. For this reason, some spouses refer to that mystery time between the wait together and the ride home as the "blackout period"—a NASA term used to describe a period of several minutes during which no communication between mission control and the astronaut can take place as the space vehicle returns to the atmosphere.

THE APPOINTMENT

Chapter 3 discusses a number of strategies in dealing with a breast cancer diagnosis and *initially* telling a spouse. But the experience of breast cancer is a long process that often lingers in a relationship for a lifetime, even if you're successfully treated. Many experts believe that a huge source of miscommunication is this "blackout period" when one spouse is in the doctor's office and the other is waiting outsidee.

The first rule is to avoid these kinds of blackouts and make it clear to your team of doctors that you want your significant other to be *included* in all your appointments. Breast cancer requires, as discussed in the last chapter, a series of decisions. Many of the decisions are lifestyle-centered and affect your spouse or partner and other family members.

But a spouse or partner can play a much larger role in the appointment process than simply companionship. For example:

- *Let your spouse listen with you at the appointment.* There may be times when, being the patient, you feel too emotional, overwhelmed, or spacy to take in all the information that's thrown at you. Your spouse can help do the listening (although sometimes a spouse's anxiety can interfere with what he hears, too). In any event, two listeners are always better than one. Later, you can both recap what went on and discuss the appointment in detail.
- *Let your partner/spouse help you by doing whatever he's good at.* Research, for example. If you're better at doing the research, fine; if he's better at it, let him handle that aspect. The important thing is that you both stay focused on helping each other. Many of the decisions you are faced with between appointments involve self-education. And that means doing Internet searches for more information; going to libraries or book stores; finding good support groups. If your spouse is good at finger walking and bringing home the informational goodies, let him.
- *Let your spouse ask the doctor questions, too.* Your spouse may have questions you never thought to ask. This contribution to the appointment can be valuable. The more answers you get, the more equipped you are to make decisions.
- *If possible, make the appointment day a pamper day, too.* Often, doctors' appointments take up a significant portion of the day. So make a day of it. Have a nice lunch before or after the appointment. Take in an afternoon movie. Get some together time that doesn't revolve around cancer. On the flip side, of course, many patients find the appointment day an anxious time. It brings up memories of the diagnosis and treatment. So acknowledge that you may feel worse than usual when this day rolls around, and allow yourself to have comfort, comfort foods, friends, and quiet support.
- *Let your spouse take care of the details on appointment day, arranging for childcare or carpooling, doing small errands such as groceries, and so on.*

LOVING A WOMAN WITH BREAST CANCER

Breast cancer changes relationships. When a woman is going through breast cancer, feelings of inadequacy and fear of losing her spouse or partner are natural reactions. Especially if a mastectomy is involved. Even when a spouse continuously reassures you by saying, "I love you," this is often not enough for the ill partner. (Although it's always nice to hear!) Are there other things a spouse can do to really reassure the ill partner? Absolutely!

OTHER WAYS TO SAY "I LOVE YOU"

What strategies have worked for other spouses facing breast cancer, and what it is it that women need from their partners during this time?

1. *Become the homemaker without asking.* Look after as many of the meals, chores, and so on as you can. Sick people often have trouble asking for help and worry about how to get everything done. Your becoming the homemaker automatically takes away the responsibility from the ill partner and makes it easier for her to rest without guilt.
2. *Random acts of romance.* Whether it's impulsively taking a day off to go to the zoo, planning a romantic weekend away, or giving your spouse a rose for every appointment she made it through, these are small things that show caring and thought and say, "I think about you when you're not around. I want to take you away from this. I want to be with you."
3. *Go to a support group.* Whether it's a "just for spouses" support group or a couples' group, go. This says: "I want to share the experience with you. I want to meet other people in the same situation so we can form meaningful friendships." One husband recounted that the most valuable experience he and his wife shared was a breast cancer support group meeting held at their home. The husband had an opportunity to listen to the needs of different women with breast cancer, which helped bring him and his wife together.
4. *Random acts of research.* Ask if anyone in your workplace has gone

through breast cancer herself or with his spouse? Talk with others and bring home more information. Cut out meaningful articles and pick out books you think she'd like. This says: "I think about you at work and throughout my day".

5. *Random acts of humor.* You know your spouse better than anyone. You know what would make her laugh more than anybody, too. So whether it's bringing home a favorite comedy video, Elvis "Love Me Tender" shampoo, or a "Madonna-inspired" mastectomy bra with gold studs and darts, do it for laughs. This says: "I want to cheer you up and I'm willing to do anything it takes."

6. *Set aside special time together once a day.* Breast cancer is an emotional experience that changes from day to day. Make a point of having one special time each day to check in with each other. How is she feeling today? How are you doing? How are kids the faring? Many couples find that staying in bed an extra ten to fifteen minutes each morning to hold each other and talk is a good time to do this.

7. *Let her set the pace.* The ill partner can set the pace of the day depending on how she's feeling. This doesn't mean that a spouse or partner shouldn't share his feelings but that he should take extra care to respond to what the ill partner is feeling.

8. *Support her if she wants to talk about the breast cancer with your friends.* People have different ways of coping, and some really choose to be more open about their illness. So if she wishes to talk about her cancer, don't feel as though you have to hide the fact that breast cancer is in your house. As discussed in Chapter 3, this may make some friends uncomfortable, but many will become better and closer friends.

What a spouse is going through

Counselors who work with breast cancer patients regret that more research into the spouse's feelings isn't done. There are some universal feelings of anxiety and angst a spouse will go through. Awareness and acknowledgment that you're not alone in having these feelings is the first step in coping with them:

- *Sleeplessness.* Waking up at two in the morning in a panic about the breast cancer is a common experience. Sharing this problem with your ill partner as well as with a counselor is a healthy way of dealing with it.
- *Separation anxiety.* You may suddenly have a tremendous need to spend more time with the ill partner and miss her terribly when she's not with you. This is a normal reaction when you're facing a life-threatening illness.
- *Not wanting to talk about your feelings.* This is most common with male partners, who our culture teaches to cope with feelings by burying them. "Take it like a man" is one piece of advice that doesn't work here. As one husband said: "If you don't talk, it still won't go away!" Going to spousal support groups where you can meet other men in the same situation is the best way to cope with this.
- *Feeling that she's "wallowing" in her cancer.* A woman going through breast cancer may want to talk about it openly—over and over again, re-hashing discussions you had yesterday, last week, or last month. You may feel as though it's not necessary to keep discussing the cancer or the treat-ment, but it is by constantly discussing it that many women integrate the experience. Be patient. When a woman does this, it's also a sign that she feels close enough to you to share.
- *Feeling left out.* In other words, friends and acquaintances will begin to call in after surgery (one breast cancer patient refers to this as the "Christmas card list" calling to check in) to see how the ill partner is doing, completely ignoring the spouse's feelings. This can lead a spouse to feel ig-nored, resentful, and unappreciated for all the caregiving he's doing. Sharing these feelings with the ill partner or a counselor is the best way to work through it.
- *Feeling differently about sex.* This is extremely normal and is discussed in detail further on, pages 195–198.

Wanting to rescue the breast

Breast cancer confronts the very sexuality of a couple, and for that reason, sex-ual partners of women diagnosed with breast cancer may have irrational wishes regarding treatment. For instance, many spouses concentrate on the end-appearance of the breasts rather than the overall cure rate of one treatment over another. This can make the decision-making process all the more stressful.

So if a doctor offers a choice of lumpectomy over a modified mastectomy, making it clear that a modified mastectomy in this situation is a more thorough surgery, a partner may sacrifice the security of that thoroughness in order to keep the breast. How should a woman react to this? With compassion. It's important in this situation for a woman to make it clear to her partner that salvaging the breast is just as important to her, but that, like her, the partner needs to grieve for the breast and let it go. In these situations, counseling is highly recommended. A good oncology counselor can help couples face the loss of the breast together, because the breast belongs to the spouse, too.

Certainly, many partners do *not* react this way, but it's still important to allow a partner the opportunity to express a sense of loss over the breast. No matter how much you deny it, the breast has played an integral role in your sexuality as a couple up until now. Grieving for the breast is discussed on page 196.

WHEN A SPOUSE LEAVES

This is the worst fear of a breast cancer patient realized: the loss of her spouse along with her breast. But it does happen from time to time in both heterosexual and same-sex relationships, what Susan Love, M.D., refers to as "jerks of both gender."

The most important piece of information this action reveals is that the relationship was not founded on sturdy ground to begin with. Spouses who do not take you in sickness were probably not that supportive when you were in health either. You just never thought about it, or you were living a compromise that worked well enough before the breast cancer but not after. The takeaway message from this is that breast cancer does not cause spouses to leave; it brings up the curtain on the relationship and shines a harsh light on it. Had you been in a car accident, a fire, or raped, this probably would have also ended the relationship.

Oddly, women who lose friends and lovers over breast cancer find it a curious blessing. On the one hand, they are lonely and depressed about it; on the other, they are glad they found out what kind of person that friend or lover really was.

Finding a good counselor to share your feelings of inadequacy and loss is imperative in this situation. Joining support groups is also recommended because being with women in the same situation can help. And, of course, surrounding yourself with supportive friends and family is in order.

MAKING LOVE AGAIN

Resuming a sex life after or during breast cancer treatment can be an emotionally and physically painful process for both of you. But couples who have been through it say it has some difficult but necessary steps that, in the long run, make the sexual road less bumpy.

DON'T SAY "IT DOESN'T MATTER"

After a mastectomy, it is noble to tell a woman that her appearance "doesn't matter," that you "love her anyway," or that you "don't care about the breast—you care about *her*." But you both know this is a lie. And it does more damage in the long run.

Breast cancer survivors and counselors highly recommend being honest about your feelings. That doesn't mean saying, as one spouse apparently did, "You're ugly now," but saying, "I loved the breast, too" or "I miss it, too" will not only validate what the woman is feeling herself, but will give the breast a place of value in your life as a couple. It had been caressed and kissed, looked at and admired, and perhaps even nurtured your children. How can it suddenly have no value to your spouse at all? It was something beautiful that you both lost. And it's a loss that you need to acknowledge together. Women whose spouses went the noble route unanimously say it made things worse because they felt alone in the grieving process.

Grieving for the losses of breast cancer

Breast cancer brings up many feelings of loss. There is not only loss of the breast, but a loss of body integrity, a loss of good health, and a loss of a "safe life." Don't be afraid to take time together, and separately, just to cry for the loss of the breast. And don't set a time limit on the grieving process because it doesn't work that way. In fact, grief is something that may overwhelm either of you at the oddest times—even years after the experience. It is a process similar to losing a family member. Smells, tastes, music, or places may suddenly remind you of a romantic experience together and the way it was before. This is normal and needs to be accepted as a normal process. Talk about the memories together and share the grief. The only way you can accept the new chest, reconstructed or not, is to give the old one a proper burial and memorial.

Touching the scars

A common experience in bed after breast cancer is for the partner to touch you everywhere but at the mastectomy site. If you have a breast left, huge amounts of attention are paid to the remaining breast while the other side is treated as a forbidden zone.

Survivors and counselors stress the importance of welcoming the mastectomy site as part of the sexual experience. Touching and caressing the site, even if it is numb, is a crucial step in reawakening your sexual experience together. Of course, there will be times when the area may be sensitive: particularly during radiation therapy or after a reconstruction surgery.

THE PRESSURE FOR RECONSTRUCTION

As discussed in Chapter 5, there are numerous decisions to be made about breast reconstruction. But the cardinal rule is to do it because you want it, not because of pressure from a partner. While many partners feel more anxious about subjecting you to more surgery after a mastectomy than about having the breast restored, many women still want reconstruction to "correct" their sex life. This is a valid reason so long as you're doing it for yourself, not because the reconstruction is some sort of condition for sexual relations that your partner has placed upon you.

But what if it is? If it is, it reveals that your partner is not coping well with your breast cancer. Instead of freaking out, make another condition: You will consider reconstruction only if your partner goes for counseling.

WHEN YOU DON'T FEEL SEXUAL BUT YOUR PARTNER DOES

The most caring and sensitive partner may not be able to make up for the fact that you feel unattractive and wholly un-sexy about your body. There are, of course, many women who will be in menopause as a result of their treatment (see Chapter 4) and may be experiencing real physical changes such as vaginal dryness, loss of libido due to hormonal changes, as well as depression, which can partly be attributed to a loss of estrogen. In one California study, a third of all breast cancer survivors reported sexual problems. About 37 percent of women surveyed said that the cancer had a negative impact on their life, while 53 percent reported that all of the changes in their body made them feel sexually un-attractive. With respect to specific physical problems, 68 percent reported problems with vaginal lubrication and 24 percent said that at least half the time, they found sex painful.

Expanding the sexual experience is an important step when re-establishing your sex life. In other words, sex does not have to equal intercourse all the time. Sensual massage, holding, and hugging, as well as experimenting with mastur-bating your partner (when you don't feel like an orgasm yourself), can substi-tute for intercourse until more emotional and physical healing takes place.

Unfortunately, because you have had breast cancer, you should not be tak-ing estrogen replacement therapy, which would take care of your menopausal symptoms. Many doctors prescribe a vaginal cream with estrogen that re-lieves dryness during intercourse. While this is still a form of estrogen, it is not very potent and is not the same thing as having estrogen in your bloodstream. Vaginal moisturizers and lubricants can also help with dryness. For more in-formation on menopause, consult Chapter 13 of my book, *The Gynecological Sourcebook*.

AVOIDING INTIMACY

Couples who have gone through breast cancer acknowledge that avoiding intimacy is one of the tricks couples use to avoid the pain of re-establishing contact. This is particularly so when the ill partner is back in commission again. One of two scenarios takes place. In the first scenario, the ill partner is feeling better and busies herself with so many things, she just "never has time" for sex anymore. She's in bed late, is exhausted, and gets up early to start her day.

In the second scenario, the well partner is so relieved that the ill partner is taking over her role in the household again, he wants to forget about the cancer and tries to put it behind them, never wanting to discuss the experience again. This greatly interferes with the couple's intimacy.

If these scenarios sound familiar, take a tip from couples who have been through it. They recommend:

- Spending more "slowed down" time together. That means going to bed earlier at night or staying in bed later in the mornings to talk and cuddle or going for more walks, and so on.
- If the ill partner (who is now well) is spending too much time away from the well partner, he should let her know that she is missed.
- Making dates with each other: lunch dates, dinner dates, and so on. Courtship is an important part of re-establishing intimacy.
- The ill partner should take care to check in with the well partner to see how he is feeling.

FERTILITY AFTER BREAST CANCER

This is a concern for younger couples who are experiencing breast cancer and haven't yet had their families. If you're having chemotherapy, there are a number of decisions you may wish to consider to maximize your fertility.

Although in most cases, the loss of fertility may be a concern that is secondary to the potential loss of one's life, there are a few options you can consider if you want very much to retain the possibility of having your own biological child. Depending on your situation, none of these options may be possible or feasible, and the risks connected with each option may not be clearly ascertainable. Still, many women feel better for asking about them.

- Discuss the idea of having your eggs harvested for an IVF procedure with your partner's sperm. Embryos can be frozen (known as cryopreservation) and transferred back into either your own uterus when you're well again or a host uterus if you're in menopause after chemotherapy. In the near future, freezing oocytes (eggs) may also become a realistic option (it is currently in its experimental stage).
- After treatment, consider pregnancy as soon as it is medically safe. Usually, you'll be cautioned to wait two years after chemotherapy before you get pregnant. Depending on your dosage of chemotherapy, ovarian function may resume for a few years before menopause sets in. Try to get pregnant as soon as your doctor considers it safe. Or, if you're not married and are not in a position to have a child yet, you may want to consider having your eggs mixed with donor sperm for future embryos or frozen (when the procedure becomes available) for a later time in your life, just in case ovarian function shuts down earlier.

For more information on assisted reproductive technology (ART) procedures, consult my book, *The Fertility Sourcebook*.

GETTING PREGNANT AFTER BREAST CANCER

Some women can get pregnant after breast cancer treatment. The concern about pregnancy after breast cancer centers on the fact that the increased hormonal levels of pregnancy might activate any latent cancer, especially if the cancer was estrogen-receptor positive. However, recent studies have suggested that pregnancy has no effect on recurrence after breast cancer treatment. All these considerations must be weighed against your desire to have a child. In the past, many younger women with intact ovaries were counseled to wait five years before they got pregnant. But since chemotherapy may cause you to have an earlier menopause, five years may be too late. The older you are when you have your chemotherapy, the more likely you are to enter permanent menopause. More aggressive drugs or longer courses of therapy can also increase your chance of entering permanent menopause. For example, a 38-year-old woman on a gentler drug has about 65 percent chance of resuming fertility after treatment, but a 44-year-old on a more aggressive drug has only a 40 percent chance of resuming fertility. Waiting two years is now the guideline because many recurrences happen in that time frame. In addition, this gives time for the chemotherapy drugs to pass through your body completely. Sometimes, however, even two years may seem too long. In this case, it is important to discuss the risks with both a medical oncologist and an obstetrician. Depending on how advanced your breast cancer was at diagnosis, a valid concern is your own mortality: will you be around to raise your child?

For what it's worth, to date, studies do not show any difference in the survival rates of women who get pregnant after breast cancer, compared with non-pregnant breast cancer survivors. But then, not many studies have been done in this area. Experts do feel that women who have had several positive nodes at the time of diagnosis have a higher risk of recurrence after pregnancy. This may or may not affect your decision about pregnancy, however.

· · · · · · ·

This chapter should not replace counseling or spousal support groups. It is merely an ice-breaker that touches the myriad of complex emotions couples face together during the breast cancer experience. The greatest fear that spouses have, of course, is losing the ill partner. This is a fear that both of you must face when the issues of recurrence and spreading confront your lives. The next chapter discusses some other ways that may make coping with breast cancer easier.

CHAPTER 7

ALL ABOUT COMPLEMENTARY MEDICINE

If you had walked into an oncologist's office in 1986 and said that you wanted to look into naturopathy in addition to your regular cancer treatment, you might have been laughed at, yelled at, or even referred to a psychiatrist for having truly "lost it." Today, things are quite different: Many oncologists will openly suggest alternative medicine to you! And even if they don't, they will encourage you to seek out other forms of healing. That is how dramatically complementary medicine has affected cancer therapy in North America. Or, more to the point, that's how dramatically cancer patients are affecting oncologists' attitudes. And that's why the term *alternative* medicine in cancer therapy has been replaced with the term *complementary* medicine.

This chapter is not meant to replace the thorough texts on alternative/ complementary medicine that are available (check the resource list at the back of this book), but is designed as a consumer's guide, if you will, to the various kinds of complementary healing available to you. If you're like me, you may know about some of the more popular routes such as Chinese herbal medicine or homeopathy, but you may not know, for example, about ayurveda or iridology. So, I'll discuss each tradition alphabetically. In addition, I will cover the basic philosophies behind several of these traditions which, though different, are alike in one respect: they all have a systemic (bodywide) approach to treatment.

THE QI TO LIFE

All ancient non-Western cultures, be they native North American, Indian, Chinese, Japanese, or Greek, believed that there were two fundamental aspects of the human body: the actual physical shell (the corporeal body) that makes cells, blood, tissue, and so on and the energy flow that makes the physical body come alive—the life force or life energy. In fact, so central to human function is this life force considered, that all non-Western cultures have a word for it: in China, it is called *chi* or *qi* (pronounced chee); in India it's called *prana*; in Japan it's called *ki*; while the ancient Greeks called it *pneuma*, which has become a prefix in medical terms having to do with breath and lungs.

While Western medicine concentrates on the corporeal body (it does not recognize the presence of a life force), non-Western, ancient healing believes that the life force heals the corporeal body, not the other way around.

Non-Western healers look upon the parts of the body as "windows" or "maps" to the body's health. In China, the ears are a complex map, with each point on the ear representing a different organ and a different part of the psyche. In reflexology (discussed further on), it is the feet which are read, since it is believed that feet can tell much about the rest of the body and the spirit. Ayurveda reads the tongue, while other traditions read the iris of the eyes, or other parts of the body. Western medicine, on the other hand, looks at every individual part for symptoms of disease and treats each part individually. So, if you went to an eye doctor with a problem of blurred vision, you would be given a prescription for glasses and sent on your way. But a Chinese doctor would tell you that the degeneration of the eyes points to an unhealthy liver, since the Chinese believe that the eyes are a direct window to the liver. (Interestingly, it is the eyes that turn yellow when one has jaundice.) The Chinese healer would then look into the causes of the liver imbalance and ask you questions about your personal relationships, your diet, your emotional well-being, and your job. The treatment may involve a host of dietary changes, stress-relieving exercises, and herbal remedies. An ayurvedic doctor may read the tongue to arrive at the same diagnosis, liver imbalance, and his approach is the same as the Chinese healer's: He, too, will ask you about your diet, lifestyle, work habits, and so on. In other words, non-Western traditions do not see the body as separate from the self. To a non-Western healer, what makes us who we are basically has to do with our individual personalities and our societal roles; who we marry, where we work, and how we feel about these things are just as important as our medical problems.

THE ANECDOTE

You know the story. Jane is given six months to live. Jane abandons Western medicine and seeks spriritual healing. Perhaps she decides to fill her life with humor and laughter; perhaps she seeks to heal herself through meditation. Six months later, she's alive and well, and her puzzled oncologist tells her that her cancer has vanished, her tumors have shrunk, her body seems for the moment to be cancer-free. What happened? Nobody knows. Jane will tell you she has healed herself. Her oncologist will say it is one of those freak things one sees every now and again that makes one realize how little one truly understands about life. Is this anecdote true? I personally know a few people who have lived this story. And I know of friends and family members who have witnessed this tale. Is this story counted as scientific proof of the spirit's power to heal the body? No, it isn't. But studies that have compared longevity rates in women who seek out other support during cancer therapy have found that breast cancer patients attending a weekly support group live twice as long as those that don't, indicating that a nurtured spirit is a potent tool in healing.

HEALING CANCER NON-WESTERN STYLE

The example about blurred vision represents the difference in approach between non-Western and Western healers. A non-Western healer would treat cancer the same way as he would the vision problem. Except in this case, it's not your liver that's believed to be in trouble, or even your breast—it is your immune system.

If you went to your family doctor with a runny nose, sneezing, and watery eyes, you would be encouraged to treat the symptoms with cough suppressants, medicines that clear your nasal passages, and so on. Not when you go to a non-Western healer. The non-Western healer will say, "You've got a cold— good! That's your body's way of eliminating waste products and toxins. Go with it. Rest, and keep sneezing." In other words, a cold is considered to be the body's way of restoring its balance.

If ridding the body of toxins restores balance, what happens when those toxins build up? Well, a variety of illnesses can develop, ranging from heart disease to cancer. Toxins are usually contained in the food we eat and the air we breathe (see Chapter 1). But non-Western healers also see certain societal roles as "toxic" and believe they can have devastating effects on the immune system. This societal toxin is stress. Hans Selye, who pioneered research into the effects of stress on the body, concluded that in our primitive states, we either confront stress or run away from it—we can either kill the attacking dog or run from it. To stay and be attacked goes against every evolutionary and human instinct. Yet most of us do this every day. Take the scenario of a child being abused by a parent. The child would like to tell the parent to stop the abuse, but can't. The child would like to run away, but can't. So the child takes the abuse. The same scenario is played out in less dramatic circumstances in the workplace. We'd like to confront the boss or quit our jobs half the time, but don't. We stay and take the abuse. This is when stress is said to have "accumulated effects" on the body, causing disease or impairing the body's ability to fight off disease. Stress can be played out in a variety of bodily "forums"—hormones (women stop menstruating under great stress, men stop producing sperm or become impotent); respiration (stress is often the trigger for asthma attacks or hyperventilation); the cardiovascular system (according to Deepak Chopra, more heart attacks occur on Monday mornings at 9:00 A.M. than at any other time); and so on.

So when your immune system is ill, be it with cancer or AIDS, a non-Western healer will attempt to heal the immune cells by invigorating them with positive thoughts, meditation, visualization, and, most importantly, by eliminating stress. Much has been written about the benefits of having a positive attitude. Norman Cousins was able to greatly prolong his life simply through laughter. We now know that smiling actually changes mood and brain chemistry, while laughter improves hormonal function, respiration, and heart function.

Eliminating toxins may also involve changing or supplementing diet; movement (through healing massages, acupuncture, and various exercises to invigorate the body); and smells (through aromatherapy, for example).

YOU CAN HAVE YOUR HERBS AND SURGERY, TOO

If non-Western medicine practices sound appealing to you, count yourself among the millions of North Americans who currently seek out complementary/alternative medicine or, rather, non-Western therapies. The good news is that non-Western healing can be beautifully combined with Western treatments for breast cancer. So you don't have to trade in one set of values for another; you can include both and form a more complete therapy—and *complete* is the root word of *complementary*.

In fact, many of the drugs we use in Western therapy, including chemotherapy agents, are actually made from herbs or plants anyway. According to Andrew Weil, a physician and author of several natural medicine books, Europeans have been complementing herbs with conventional drugs for a long time. In Germany, doctors routinely prescribe herbal remedies for a host of health problems such as colds and even depression. In fact, a herb called Saint John's wort, with the active ingredient hypericin, is a popular antidepressant in Germany.

Most people don't realize that roughly 25 percent of all pharmaceutical products come from natural plants. Morphine and codeine are derived from the opium poppy, while the anti-cancer drugs vincristine and vinblastine come from periwinkle. Even aspirin comes from the salicin in willow bark. To date, at least sixteen herbs have been approved by the Food and Drug Administration, which allows the manufacturers of these herbs to make claims on labeling and to sell them over the counter.

ARE THERE RISKS?

Out of the roughly six hundred herbs available in the United States (less are available in Canada), less than twelve have been tested in scientifically controlled trials to determine whether they are safe and work better than a placebo. About fifty herbs have been tested under more lax conditions.

As of this writing, the American Herbal Products Association, a trade group of herbal manufacturers, is compiling a reference manual on six hundred herbal ingredients, which includes directions for safe use. Some experts suggest comparing herbs to coffee when weighing dosage: two cups of coffee per day is considered safe; five cups may cause headaches and nervousness; fifteen cups can cause serious side effects.

It's important to keep in mind that when it comes to researching alternative therapies, most Western researchers don't know enough about them to design proper studies. And, many of these ancient disciplines don't lend themselves well to Western-style research such as double-blind controlled studies.

For now, so long as your Western doctors know what your Eastern doctors are doing, and vice versa, complementary medicine can help to optimize your standard cancer treatment. The danger arises when you don't disclose the other therapies you are using to your Western practitioners, or you decide, for example, not to have surgery for an early-stage, highly treatable, and curable breast cancer, instead opting for acupuncture only. This situation differs from the case of someone with advanced metastatic disease who decides not to have chemotherapy and opts for homeopathy. In the first case, cancer can be absolutely cured through Western techniques, while overall health can be strengthened through non-Western techniques. In the second case, there is no certain cure in either tradition, so strengthening the body and mind to help fight the cancer is a perfectly logical approach.

There are other risks with non-Western medicine that you should be aware of:

1. There is no scientific proof to support the claims or the efficacy of most of the treatments you'll be offered.
2. Since there is no advisory board or set of guidelines governing non-Western practitioners, the alternative industry attracts quacks and charlatans, and the cost of some therapies may be exhorbitant.

3. Academic credentials are all over the map in this industry. Again, beware humbugs.

4. Certain preparations are boiled down in clay or metal pots, leaving residues of lead, mercury, arsenic, gold, or cadmium. There have also been reports that sometimes Chinese herbal preparations are laced with prescription drugs. You have to be careful and purchase your preparations from reputable places.

5. Dosages are all over the map. The active ingredient in many herbs may not be accurately measured. One reason modern medicine moved away from herbal preparations is that the drugs were easier to purify and standardize. When you buy ten 325 mg tablets of a painkiller, that's what you get. But when you buy ten capsules of a herb, the dosages may vary from capsule to capsule.

6. Sometimes you're blamed for a treatment's failure—apparently, your body would have responded if your mind had been more "open." Don't you dare fall for this nonsense.

7. Some non-Western healers may coerce you into dropping out of Western therapy even when you're clearly responding to it. This is not ethical behavior.

8. You may prefer to abandon clearly curative Western therapies in favor of non-Western therapy. This can have truly unfortunate consequences.

FINDING ETHICAL AND QUALIFIED HEALERS

First, do some homework on the type of tradition that attracts you. Use this chapter as a guide to more thorough sources on the various traditions available. Then, use your "hairdresser" rules to find non-Western healers: Go to people recommended by other cancer patients, your oncologists, friends, or acquaintances. If that's not possible, there are academic institutes for various traditions that can recommend accredited healers in the discipline you want to try out. Keep in mind that there may not be anyone practicing the kind of medicine you want in the area you live in. You may need to travel to an urban center for your treatment.

Insurance coverage

Insurance companies are starting to cover complementary medicine. Several companies such as Prudential pay for acupuncture for chronic pain, while Blue Cross of Washington and Alaska allows you to choose from a group of acupuncturists, homeopaths, and naturopaths for an extra $176 a year. One of the best plans is available through American Western Life, based in Foster City, California. In addition to standard coverage, it pays for acupuncture, ayurvedic medicine, biofeedback, massage, and hypnotherapy, and the policyholder pays just $10 per visit. American Western policies are available in Arizona, California, Colorado, New Mexico, and Utah, but it is reported to have plans for expansion in Hawaii, Illinois, Michigan, Oregon, and Washington.

If you don't have insurance coverage, experts suggest the following:

1. Get your doctor to prescribe the complementary therapy you want. Many plans will cover you if you have a doctor's prescription.
2. If your doctor is not open to this, you could ask your alternative practitioner to suggest a doctor who is willing to prescribe the therapy—for insurance coverage purposes—but don't abandon your oncologist just for this reason!
3. The IRS has ruled that both acupuncture and chiropractic care are legitimate medical deductions.
4. Pester your insurance company for coverage by calling its benefits administrator. You can negotiate coverage—it's done all the time.

THE A TO Z OF COMPLEMENTARY MEDICINE

Following is a brief explanation of the types of complementary medicine available. Again, you're encouraged to go to more detailed sources after you've been through this overview.

ACUPUNCTURE

This is an ancient Chinese healing art that aims to restore the smooth flow of life energy, or *qi*, in your body. Acupuncturists believe that your *qi* can be accessed from various points on your body, such as your ear, for example. Each point is also associated with a specific organ. So, if your physical health permits, an acupuncturist will use a fine needle on a very specific point to restore *qi* to various organs. Each of the roughly two thousand points on your body has a specific therapeutic effect when stimulated. The National Institutes of Health (NIH) is funding research that studies the effects of acupuncture on depression, attention-deficit disorder, hypersensitivity disorder, osteoarthritis, and postoperative dental pain. One large study found that acupuncture offered short-term relief for 50 to 80 percent of patients with acute or chronic pain. It is now believed that acupuncture stimulates the release of endorphins, which is why it is effective at reducing pain. Also, cancer patients on the drug cisplatin experienced less nausea when given acupuncture.

What it complements

In cancer therapy, acupuncture is used for pain management either after surgery or during chemotherapy or radiation treatment. It has also been used in operating rooms to control pain.

AYURVEDIC MEDICINE

Ayurveda is an ancient Indian approach to health and wellness that has stood the test of time. This three-thousand-year-old philosophy essentially divides the universe into three basic constitutions or energies known as *doshas*. The three *doshas* are based on wind *(vata)*, fire *(pitta)*, and earth *(kapha)*. These *doshas* govern our bodies, personalities, and activities. One person may be predominantly *kapha*—thicker in build, often overweight, and more lethargic—another may be predominantly *vata*—thinner in build, usually with a more finicky appetite, and a more hyperactive personality. When our *doshas* are balanced, all functions well; when they are not balanced, a state of disease (dis-ease or not at ease) can set in. Restoring the balance involves changing your diet to suit your predominant *dosha* (foods are classified as *kapha, vata,* or *pitta*); doing certain yoga exercises; practicing meditation; and incorporating certain lifestyle habits.

Ayurveda places a great deal of emphasis on good digestion and elimination. If these two processes are not in harmony, we can suffer from a variety of health problems, ranging from bad breath and headaches (both caused by constipation) to more serious diseases such as cancer.

An ayurvedic doctor will determine your constitution by your appearance, lifestyle habits, and overall personality traits. In addition, the tongue is considered a "map" of the organs that implicates which part of the body is imbalanced. The NIH is funding research into the use of ayurvedic treatment for Parkinson's disease.

What it complements

Life in general. This is a comprehensive approach to life, which can be used whether or not you have cancer.

CHELATION

Popular among people with clogged arteries or heart disease, this is not used for cancer treatment, but I'm including it here because you may have heard about chelation (prounounced key-lay-tion) and been confused about what it is. Chelation refers to the use of agents to remove toxic metals (such as lead and cadmium) and excess copper and iron from the body. The belief is that the accumulation of heavy metals in the body is the cause of circulatory problems such as atherosclerosis.

Therapy involves the drug ethylene diamine tetracetic acid (EDTA), which is supposed to help clear the blood vessels. Chelation therapy is supposed to restore blood flow to every part of the body (it was initially used for lead poisoning). To date, no studies on chelation therapy have been done; its practitioners complain that this is because appropriate funding has not been allocated.

What it complements

Clogged arteries rather than cancer per se.

CHINESE MEDICINE

About three thousand years old, Chinese medicine, like ayurvedic medicine, bases the universe on two constitutions, yin and yang. Everything—be it temperaments, organs, foods, activities, or individual personalities—is yin or yang. Yang is considered a male constitution, while yin is believed to be female. But both yin and yang co-exist in all individuals. In addition to yin and yang, there are five elements (similar to *doshas* in ayurvedic medicine) based on fire, earth, wood, metal and water, to which different organs in our bodies correspond. Like ayurveda, Chinese medicine is based on the belief that when everything is balanced, the body is healthy and the life force *(qi)* flows uninterrupted; without balance, *qi* can be disturbed, and disease can set in. Finding the balance is thus the goal of Chinese medicine. Balance is restored through diet, which is either adjusted or supplemented with herbs; through the stimulation of pressure points on the body with acupuncture (which is part of Chinese medicine); or through massage. Lifestyle may require changing as well.

What it complements

Life in general. Again, this is an all-encompassing approach to life, and can be used whether or not you have cancer.

CHIROPRACTIC MEDICINE

This is becoming much more accepted in Western practice, but your health insurer will still consider it alternative therapy.

The word *chiropractic* comes from the Greek *chiro* and *prakrikos,* which means "done by hand." The tradition was perfected in the late 1800s by Daniel David Palmer of Port Perry, Ontario. Palmer was a self-taught healer who eventually founded a practice in Iowa. He believed that all drugs were harmful and that disease is caused by vertebrae impinging on spinal nerves.

According to chiropractors, the brain sends energy to every organ along the nerves running through the spinal cord. When the vertebrae of the spinal column get displaced due to stress, poor posture, and so on, this can interfere with or block normal nerve transmission (interferences are known as subluxations). In order to cure disease in the body, the chiropractor must remove the interference or blockages. This is done through adjustments such as quick thrusts, massage, and pressure along the spinal column. This is believed to move the spinal vertebrae back to its normal position.

Adjustments sometimes involve manipulating the head and extremities (elbows, ankles, knees). This is generally done by hand, but chiropractors can use special devices to aid them in treatment, as well.

A chiropractor will take your medical history, do a general physical exam (the manual exam may also help to catch tumors along the spine), and may X ray your spine to look for malalignments. Don't allow an X ray to be done until your oncologist clears it—you've probably had a lot of radiation already. In addition to giving you a spinal adjustment, chiropractors also counsel you on exercise, heat treatment, and nutrition.

What it complements

Most people go to a chiropractor for help in managing back pain, but many find it is a great stress reliever as well. During cancer therapy, a chiropractor can help to alleviate the pain and stress associated with various treatments such as surgery pain.

ENVIRONMENTAL MEDICINE

This is still considered alternative medicine, even though it should probably be incorporated into conventional practice. Environmental medicine is currently a sub-specialty of the field of allergy and immunology, sometimes called clinical ecology. An environmental medicine practitioner will look at the impact of environmental factors on your health, particularly focusing on foods, chemicals, water, and pesticides, as well as indoor and outdoor air quality. Treatment usually involves cleaning up whatever is affecting you; if the problem is air quality, you might need to move or simply install air filters, for example). Sometimes drugs are used to treat specific allergies, but only in minimal doses.

HERBAL THERAPY

Herbal therapy is discussed separately because you don't need to go to any one healer for herbs; they can be found in abundance in health food stores and plant nurseries. And, besides, books and newspaper health columns flood us with information about herbs.

One native North American tribe believes that disease was given to humans by animals in an effort to even out the odds for survival, but the plant kingdom had a meeting in which they decided that they would do their best to cure disease and make themselves available for preventive and curative remedies.

Every culture in the world has relied on plants and herbs to treat illness. The Sumerians were using herbal therapies as early as 4000 B.C. By 3000 B.C., the Chinese were using over one thousand medicinal herbs.

Herbs are widely used in Western medicine as well. About 25 percent of all prescription drugs in North America are derived from plants. Half the chemotherapy drugs used to treat cancer today come from natural herb or plant sources. They are available in health food stores and pharmacies—these herbs are effective, but can sometimes be harmful if they contain toxic metals or other dangerous substances. Herbal medicine is becoming popular because people are realizing that over-the-counter or prescription drugs are often no more or less potent than herbal remedies. So why not go more natural?

Much like the pharmaceutical drugs of today, herbal therapies became established through trial and error (of course, the same could be said for magic spells). Alternative medicine practitioners argue that pharmaceutical companies don't fund research into herbal therapies because these remedies are natural and hence cannot be patented.

In the United States, over $880 million of herbs and vitamins have been sold every year since about 1993. Plant drugs are classified as food or food additives in the United States, so many herbs are sold in grocery and health food stores, besides pharmacies. Canada classifies drugs differently and only allows the sale of drugs that have received a drug identification number—something many herbs do not have. Herbs that cannot be found in pharmacies can be found in health food stores or Chinese herb stores. But a few natural products are actually banned in Canada, including melatonin.

What it complements
Conventional Western treatments for all illnesses. Make sure you tell your doctor which herbs you are taking. Bring in the bottle so your doctor can read the label and ingredients.

HOLISTIC MEDICINE
Holistic medicine started as a reaction to the rather narrow body-focused approach of Western medicine. A holistic doctor looks at the whole person: body, mind, and spirit. A variety of Western and non-Western techniques are used in treatment. Essentially, a holistic doctor enters into a partnership with the patient, encouraging the patient to learn how to reduce risks of illness and how to choose therapies that the patient is comfortable with. It is an approach to health that emphasizes self-care and personal responsibility for wellness.

What it complements
All Western therapies.

HOMEOPATHY
This approach began in the early nineteenth century as a reaction to the "heroic measures" commonly used then to treat disease. These heroic measures included bloodletting, induced vomiting, and massive doses of drugs. Pioneered by Dr. Samuel Hahnemann, a German physician who was trained in conventional medicine and chemistry but was disillusioned with conventional approaches to disease, homeopathy is based on the theory that "like cures like," or what Hahnemann called the Law of Similars. Essentially, a substance that produces certain symptoms in a healthy person is believed to cure a sick person

with the same symptoms. He coined the term *homeopathy* from the Greek *homoios* and *pathos* (similar sickness).

To treat disease, a homeopath uses minute doses of substances. Hahnenman found he could preserve the healing properties and eliminate side effects of a medication through a pharmacological process he called "potentization," in which substances are diluted with distilled water. The more diluted a substance, the more potent Hahnenman found it to be. As a result of this discovery, he formulated the controversial Law of Infinitesimals, which basically means that good things come in small quantities. To prove the theory, Hahneman constantly referred to the minute amounts of hormones our bodies produce—the amounts are minute but so potent that they govern our bodies.

Homeopathy was very popular in the nineteenth century for treating infectious diseases, particularly epidemics. Homeopathy is often confused with holistic medicine, but it is a different discipline. Homeopaths call their approach holistic because they believe they're treating not just one organ, but the entire patient. They see symptoms as positive signs that the body is trying to defend itself against an underlying disease. In fact, homeopathic drugs might even aggravate symptoms. A homeopath will say that a worsening of symptoms is really a sign that the body is stimulating its own self-healing mechanism.

Homeopathy involves taking a very long medical history. There are more than 2,000 remedies used by a homeopath, all derived from various plant, mineral, animal, and chemical sources. Some examples include marigold flowers, onions, graphite snake venom, honeybee extract, and other wild concoctions. At first, these treatments may sound dangerous, but since the doses are so diluted, they are widely recognized as harmless at worst in the general population.

What it complements

Since there is such an emphasis on treating ailments, it may or may not complement chemotherapy or radiation therapy. Just make sure you're straight with all your doctors about what you're on already before you take that snake venom.

IRIDOLOGY

No healer believes that the eyes are windows to the soul more than an iridologist. Iridology is not really a therapy but a diagnostic tool used by a wide variety of non-Western healers. Iridology studies changes in the texture and color of the iris and correlates these changes with the physical and mental state of health. An iridologist may not only be able to tell you about an unsuspected thyroid problem, but may also tell you that you have an unhealthy relationship with your spouse. Many people have found the experience very accurate and helpful.

Iridology is also used to identify dietary deficiencies and the accumulation of toxic chemicals in the body. In fact, just as a Western doctor may send you for an ultrasound, a natural medicine doctor may send you to an iridologist to expand a diagnosis.

Developed in the nineteenth century by Ignatz von Peczely, a Hungarian physician, iridology was adapted for modern practice in the 1950s by Bernard Jensen, an American chiropractor. Jensen based his practice on detailed diagrams of the left and right irises. He assigned every organ, many body parts, and all bodily functions to a specific location on one or both irises.

Iridologists believe that the degrees of light and darkness in the iris hold enormous clues to the body's general health. They also examine textures of fibers in the iris. Of course, ayurvedic or Chinese practitioners also examine the eyes for clues to the body's general health. Iridologists will counsel you on nutrition or life habits, but, for the most part, will send you elsewhere for treatment.

What it complements

Diagnostic tests and Western diagnoses.

MASSAGE THERAPY

A massage can be beneficial whether you receive it from your spouse or from a massage therapist trained in any one of a dozen techniques ranging from shiatsu to Swedish massage.

The *Yellow Emperor's Classic of Internal Medicine*, published in 2700 B.C. (the text that frames the entire Chinese medicine tradition), had extensive references to massage. Chinese medicine in fact recommends massage as a treatment for a variety of illnesses.

Swedish massage, the technique Westerners are are familiar with, was developed in the nineteenth century by a Swedish doctor and poet, Per Henrik, who borrowed techniques from ancient Egypt, China, and Rome.

It is out of Swedish massage of the West and shiatsu massage of the East that all the many forms of massage grew. While the philosophies and styles of each tradition differ, their goal is the same: to mobilize the natural healing properties of the body that help it maintain or restore optimal health.

Shiatsu-inspired massage focuses on balancing the life force *(qi)*, discussed at the beginning of this chapter. Swedish-inspired massage works more on physiological principles such as relaxing muscles to improve the blood flow through connective tissues, and thus strengthening the cardiovascular system.

All massages use numerous gliding and kneading techniques along with deep circular movements and vibrations that relax muscles, improve circulation, and increase mobility. This is known to help relieve stress, and often muscle and joint pain. In fact, a number of employers include massage therapy on their health plans.

What it complements

An excellent way to combat the stress of conventional treatments, postoperative stiffness, as well as pain management in more advanced stages of cancer.

NATUROPATHY

Naturopathy encompasses a broad spectrum of natural therapies. In fact, it is now a recognized graduate degree in North America; two colleges in the United States and one in Canada grant the degree of naturopathic doctor (N.D.).

Naturopathy is not a single tradition of healing but an umbrella term that refers to an entire array of healing approaches that are based on the body's intrinsic healing powers. This tends to appeal to people who distrust prescription medications or are interested in preventive therapies.

N.D.s educate their patients about lifestyles that can lead to degenerative diseases such as osteoporosis. In many ways, an N.D.'s advice will not differ much from the advice of conventional doctors regarding low-fat, high-fiber diets, stress reduction, and so on. However, an N.D. will not recommend surgery for a precancerous tumor and will prefer to treat through nutritional changes. But when necessary, N.D.s refer patients to conventional doctors and specialists for regular medical procedures, especially for breast cancer. N.D.s attempt to instill in their patients the belief that prescription drugs are costly and encourage reliance on natural medicine, including acupuncture, herbs, hydrotherapy, homeopathy, vitamin and mineral supplements, and so on.

What it complements
Western therapy of all kinds.

REFLEXOLOGY

This is a twentieth century version of an ancient healing and relaxation technique that is probably as old, if not older, than acupuncture. Western reflexology was developed by Dr. William Fitzgerald, an American ear, nose, and throat specialist, who talked about reflexology as "zone therapy," but in fact, reflexology is practiced in several cultures, including Egypt, India, Africa, China, and Japan.

Reflexologists believe the feet are a map of the organs. The feet contain valuable pressure points that stimulate the life force. By applying pressure to certain parts of the feet, reflexologists can ease pain and tension and can restore the body's life force.

Like most Eastern healing arts, reflexology aims to release the flow of energy through the body along its various pathways. Reflexologists believe that when this energy is trapped for some reason, illness can result, and the body can begin to heal itself only when the energy is released.

A reflexologist views the foot as a microcosm of the entire body. Individual reference points, or reflex areas, on the foot correspond to all major organs, glands, and parts of body. Applying pressure to a specific area of the foot stimulates the movement of energy to the corresponding body part. Reflexologists don't limit themselves to the feet, however. They also work on hands and ears, although the feet are the most preferred site.

What it complements
Western diagnosis, therapies, and pain management.

· · · · · · ·

If you're considering complementary medicine, a good book to refer to is *Choices in Healing* by Michael Lerner, M.D. (1994, MIT Press). Many cancer specialists may not be in favor of you seeking out complementary medicine, however, although their attitude is shifting radically. In fact, many Western-trained physicians are now opening up alternative-medicine practices or incorporating certain alternative traditions into their current practice. Complementary medicine is especially popular among cancer patients facing recurrence and metastatic disease, discussed next.

CHAPTER 8

THE SECOND
TIME AROUND

I wish I didn't have to write this chapter. If you are reading it, it means you are either fearing a recurrence of breast cancer or you have been diagnosed with either a recurrence or a second primary tumor (that is, a new cancer not related to the first one).

This chapter tells you who is more likely to experience a recurrence (although much more research is needed in this area). It also discusses the difference between local recurrence (another localized tumor is found with no evidence of spread) and metastasis or metastatic disease (a spread). This chapter also takes you through the treatment options for both types of recurrence, discusses symptoms and complications that can arise, and outlines all the other options available to you.

Breast cancer survivors point out that even when one is cancer-free, one can spend the rest of one's life fearing a recurrence. In this sense, this chapter may be well worth reading because it will help prepare you to make certain decisions about lifestyle and treatment, should a recurrence happen down the road.

THE RISK OF RECURRENCE

There are three major rules that govern recurrence. First, the earlier and more localized your cancer was at "first discovery," the less likely you are to experience recurrence. Second, premenopausal women who opted for adjuvant chemotherapy and postmenopausal women who opted for hormone therapy are less likely to develop a recurrence. This has been proven in numerous large, controlled studies. Third, the longer you live cancer-free, the longer you'll continue to live cancer-free, although 25 to 30 percent of all node-negative women will have a recurrence.

Why does this happen? Well, we know that women first diagnosed with an early in situ cancer (see Chapter 3) are less likely to have a metastasis (also called distant recurrence) than women first diagnosed with invasive cancer. *But* they are still at risk for a *local* recurrence (a recurrence of the first tumor in the same breast or chest wall) or a regional recurrence (a recurrence of the cancer in the axillary lymph nodes). We also know that women with stage 1 invasive cancer (see Chapter 3) are 75 to 95 percent likely to live cancer-free for ten years or more after their initial treatment. But half of all women with stage 2 invasive cancer and 75 percent of women with advanced local tumors (this means isolated but large tumors), can expect a recurrence five to ten years after treatment.

THE SECOND TUMOR

A second tumor does not necessarily mean that your breast cancer has spread; it can be a second *primary* tumor, meaning that it is a brand new cancer that's out there on its own. Women more likely to experience second primary tumors have:

- A history of benign tumors (see Chapter 2) prior to their initial breast cancer diagnosis
- Been diagnosed with lobular carcinoma in situ (see Chapter 3)
- A family history of estrogen-dependent cancers: breast cancer, endometrial cancer, ovarian cancer, or colon cancer (see Chapter 1)

What *doesn't* make a difference to the life of a second primary tumor is your age, even though age makes a huge difference the first time around. Nor does the amount of radiation therapy you had the first time matter. This is because radiation therapy is a local treatment for breast cancer, meaning that it does not course through your body systems unlike chemotherapy, which is considered a systemic treatment. (Both radiation therapy and chemotherapy are discussed in Chapter 4).

Where can you find cancer again?

In lots of places: the breasts (even in the same breast, if you've had a partial mastectomy—this happens in roughly 10 percent of all cases of recurrence); the chest wall (if you've had a mastectomy); the lymph nodes under the arm (a.k.a. axillary lymph nodes); on the skin's surface; above the collar bone; or behind the breast bone. Recurrence sites are shown in figure 8.1.

But my doctor told me chemotherapy was insurance!

Dozens of studies on hundreds of thousands of women in numerous countries have shown that adjuvant chemotherapy and radiation therapy clearly reduce the rate of recurrence and increase survival. Nevertheless, adjuvant therapy is not a guarantee against recurrence or against a second breast cancer. It is an "insurance" in the sense that you did everything in your power to reduce the risk of recurrence. And if you had adjuvant chemotherapy, you did.

DIETARY FAT AND RECURRENCE

In the same way that dietary fat intake may influence breast cancer occurrence (see Chapter 1), it may influence recurrence, too, one hypothesis suggests. Over the last couple of years, researchers have been studying whether the reduction of fat in the diet of breast cancer patients can help prevent the cancer from coming back. A 1994 study looked at 735 women treated for stage 2 and stage 3 breast cancers and found that women who were overweight had a higher incidence of recurrence than women who were of normal weight or underweight. The general conclusion of this study was that if you're still eating a high-fat diet or are obese, you may have a greater chance of recurrence—even when you have the best medical treatments available. For fat-cutting information, see Chapter 10, pages 257–259.

ESTROGEN AND RECURRENCE

If you've been initially treated for breast cancer and your cancer was estrogen-receptor positive, you're pretty much "blacklisted" from taking estrogen in the form of either a contraceptive (if you're still having periods) or hormone replacement therapy (after menopause). In fact, any book on menopause or HRT will tell you that you need to weigh the risks of heart disease against breast cancer when you make the estrogen decision. In the past, doctors would have said that for you, there really is no decision to be made about HRT. The answer is *no*. The only exception to this rule is if your cancer was not estrogen-receptor positive, which happens in about 10 percent of cases. As discussed in Chapter 1, however, there has been some change in the HRT/breast cancer philosophy. HRT is not necessarily contraindicated. You need to discuss HRT in detail with your cancer specialist so you can weigh the pros and cons. To the majority of women, most doctors will give the option of using a vaginal cream with estrogen to lessen vaginal dryness. The amount of estrogen in these creams is considered marginal and not a real risk factor for recurrence. (See Chapter 6 for more information on fertility and sexuality, and Chapter 4 for more information on menopausal symptoms.)

If I can't have HRT, what am I supposed to do about osteoporosis and heart disease?

There are definite diet and lifestyle modifications you can make to lessen the risks of both osteoporosis and heart disease. Osteoporosis, for example, can be prevented to a large extent by increasing calcium intake and by exercising! As for heart disease, aside from genetics, there are three principal causes of heart disease in women—currently the number one killer of women. These three causes are smoking (which is the number one cause of lung cancer—a cancer that kills more women than breast cancer, by the way); obesity; and stress. So even a woman who is on HRT needs to be mindful of these risks.

A female cardiac surgeon recently told me that there is absolutely no excuse to smoke anymore, given the vast amounts of literature that tell us of the dangers. She's right. So if you smoke, stop.

If you are overweight, you are going to have a number of health risks aside from heart disease. This is because, as discussed in Chapter 1, the more fat you have on your body, the higher your estrogen levels may be. In fact, many obese women never experience any menopausal symptoms due to their high estrogen levels.

Are there any drugs I can take to reduce my cholesterol?

Interestingly, hormone therapy for breast cancer patients (former or current) offers the same LDL/HDL benefits as traditional hormone replacement therapy. Of course, there are other side effects of hormone therapy that you might not be so keen on (discussed here and in Chapter 4), but you should definitely factor in this protective effect when you make your decision.

And of course, there are a variety of cholesterol-lowering drugs your doctor can prescribe that don't interfere with a breast cancer history, although they should be prescribed only after you make some real effort to adjust your diet.

And, finally, stress. If breast cancer taught you anything, it was how to "let go" of all those trivial problems that account for so of much our day-to-day stresses. Not that breast cancer isn't stressful, but you're in a better position than most women to understand how to prioritize and concentrate on the important things, instead of trying to do everything. Every stress management book and course will recommend prioritizing and list-making as a way to cut down on the amount of activities you're doing in a given day. The books and courses will also talk about methods you may have *already* explored in coping with your initial cancer: yoga, breathing, relaxation techniques, and so on.

DETECTING RECURRENCE

Once you've undergone initial treatment for breast cancer, you will most likely become a permanent outpatient. You will need to have a mammogram done every six to twelve months on the side that had breast cancer (if you had a wide excision) and on the "cancerless" side. Once you reach the five-year cancer-free mark, an annual mammogram is acceptable for both breasts.

You will also be seeing your surgeon for manual breast exams every six months for the next five years, and annually thereafter.

If you had chemotherapy, you may also have bi-annual appointments with your medical oncologist, who will most likely manage your blood tests and imaging tests to rule out a metastasis in the bone or liver. Surgeons or primary care physicians can manage this, too. As discussed in past chapters, there is a blood test that can measure CA15-3, an antigen produced by cancer cells, which can accurately rule out recurrence 92 percent of the time. When it comes to confirming a recurrence, it's accurate only 47 percent of the time.

On your own, you should continue to do a monthly breast self-exam, discussed in Chapter 2. You should also keep a health diary, recording how you're feeling from day to day or week to week. Because there are often symptoms associated with a spreading of cancer, you must report immediately any of the symptoms outlined on page 231–232 to your doctor to rule out a recurrence.

Fears of follow-up

As discussed in Chapter 4, many oncologists are shifting their follow-up philosophy and challenging the assumption that more follow-up is better. Some oncologists may even allow follow-ups when the patient feels like it or believes she needs to. There is considerable stress involved in follow-up appointments because many women treat the follow-up as a verdict that will determine how they live until their next follow-up exam—being told "you're fine" means that you're fine only *until* the next appointment. And follow-up appointments bring up memories of the initial diagnosis and treatment. But what happens when you're told at your follow-up appointment that your cancer is back? This is why cancer specialists are now seriously looking at the stress factor involved in follow-ups.

DEALING WITH DIAGNOSIS—AGAIN!

Recurrence can mean one of two things: another localized tumor or breast cancer tumors in other parts of your body, such as your bones, lungs, liver, and so on. In the first scenario, you have what's known as a *local recurrence*. Sometimes this situation is the mirror image of what you faced the first time around. Sometimes it is a completely different scenario, in that you may have a larger or smaller tumor than the first time or may have the recurrence diagnosed at a lesser or more advanced stage. And, as discussed earlier, a second tumor can be found on the same breast or the same side as before.

When cancer is found somewhere *other* than a breast or axillary (armpit) nodes, such as the bone or lungs, this means your breast cancer is spreading or metastasizing. At this point, your breast cancer is considered more advanced— this is known as metastatic disease, which translates simply to "spread disease."

For both local recurrence and metastasis, treatment options depend on a number of factors such as:

- Your general health right now
- Your age
- Whether you've had chemotherapy or radiation therapy the first time around
- What kind of breast surgery you had the first time around
- The severity of your situation
- The odds of a cure
- Your lifestyle preferences
- Your health insurance (not a concern for Canadians as of this writing)

Whether or not you've been expecting the news, you are again urged to take time to absorb it yourself before you tell others, as well as to gather as much information about the second cancer as you can. Review the section on dealing with diagnosis and doctors in Chapter 3 for more information on questions to ask and on breaking the news to your spouse, family or friends. Chapter 3 discusses a number of strategies in detail; you may need to re-employ many of the same ones you used the first time around.

NEW QUESTIONS TO ASK

Obviously, a local recurrence is better news than metastatic disease. But in either scenario, you nezed to find out the following from your the surgeon or medical oncologist who gave you the news:

1. *How will my treatment differ from the first time around?* If you opted

against chemotherapy or hormone therapy the first time around, will you have it now, for example? Is this cancer operable by surgery? This will help you plan your life in the months to come.

2. *How much time can I take to make my decisions about treatment?* In most cases, experts urge you to take a week or two to gather more information so you can make an informed decision about treatment.

3. *What are the odds this time around?* As discussed in Chapter 3, sometimes you need to weigh poor odds against quality of life.

4. *What's the best, most realistic scenario in terms of treatment results?* If you have metastatic disease, is a cure possible, or are you looking at treating symptoms and maintaining comfort and quality of life? See Chapter 7 for more details.

5. *Where can I find other patients who are/were in the same situation?* Sometimes the best information comes from other patients who have already faced the same decisions you're making right now. What was the outcome of their decisions? Why did they make the choices they did? Seeking out other patients is an important step in gathering information.

6. *How does this recurrence change my life expectancy?* Sometimes it doesn't; sometimes it does.

7. *(For advanced cancer) Should I be looking into home care or hospice arrangements?*

8. *What about alternative or complementary medicine/therapies?* It is important to check if your surgeon and/or oncologists are open to you seeing someone outside traditional Western discipline. This is discussed in greater detail in Chapter 7.

9. *What new therapies can you offer that weren't available the first time around?* Two years in the 1990s is like ten years in the 1980s in terms of medical research. You may be able to withstand much higher doses of chemotherapy thanks to bone marrow transplant advancements, and so on.

10. *How does my age affect my treatment?* As discussed in Chapters 3 and 4, the outcome of chemotherapy and hormone therapy is different in pre- and postmenopausal women.

TREATING A LOCAL RECURRENCE

Surgery is the first option offered to you when a local recurrence is diagnosed. The kind of surgery you have this time depends on what kind of surgery you had the first time around and on which side the cancer is this time.

SIDE 1

If you have a local recurrence on the same breast as before, (I refer to this as "side 1"), you will need to have a modified radical mastectomy, if you haven't already had one. If you've already had a mastectomy on that side, the tumor will still need to come out. In addition, a preventive mastectomy for the cancer-free side 2 may be an option worth considering.

Both external and internal radiation therapy will be recommended as well. But if you've already had radiation on side 1 once, and the recurrence is at a more advanced stage, radiation may not be as wise a choice as more systemic (bodywide) therapy. If your oncologists feel a second course of radiation is of benefit, your dosage may differ, depending on how much radiation you received on side 1 the first time around. Radiation therapy is discussed in detail in Chapter 4.

Depending on the staging of your cancer this time around, if you're at high risk of developing metastatic disease, a second or even third round of chemotherapy or hormone therapy, often at higher dosages, will probably be recommended.

If you have not had chemotherapy or hormone therapy before and have received only local treatment to side 1 (this means surgery and radiation, but no medication), chemotherapy will be recommended. Chemotherapy is discussed in detail in Chapter 4.

The odds

A local recurrence on side 1 after a partial mastectomy is better news than a side 1 recurrence on the chest wall after a modified or radical mastectomy. In the second scenario, you're at a high risk of developing metastatic disease.

Figure 8.1

LOCAL AND REGIONAL RECURRENCE

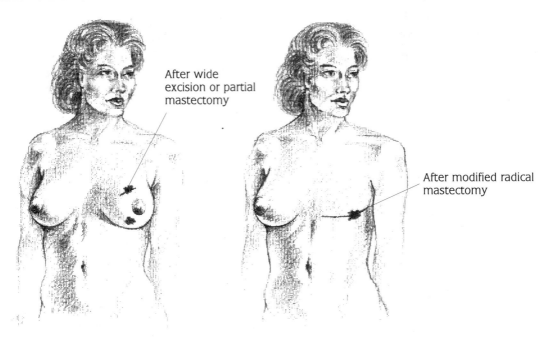

After wide
excision or partial
mastectomy

After modified radical
mastectomy

Even though you will be (re)offered chemotherapy and/or hormone therapy after more surgery, the benefits aren't clear. That's where you need to do the weighing of pros and cons.

SIDE 2

If the recurrence is on the other breast (I refer to this as "side 2"), and side 1 is still cancer-free, then the rules outlined in Chapter 3 regarding mastectomy procedures for the various stagings of breast cancer apply. However, because you've now had a recurrence, your surgeon may not be as keen on breast conserving procedures as on life-preserving procedures. In other words, your surgeon may well say "Forget it. I want that cancer out once and for all, and I think you should have a bilateral modified radical mastectomy this time." The recurrence on side 2 may be seen as a "warning" to act as aggressively as possible.

In addition, radiation to side 2 is almost a certainty, while chemotherapy and hormone therapy will again depend on what was done the first time around. Roughly 5 percent of women with cancer in one breast will develop it on the other side.

METASTATIC DISEASE

Also referred to as distant or systemic recurrence, metastatic disease means the breast cancer has spread to other organs. If breast cancer spreads to your bones or lungs, however, it doesn't suddenly become "bone cancer" or lung cancer"— it remains breast cancer in those sites.

Breast cancer cells use the blood stream or lymphatic systems as transit systems to get to other parts of the body. As for the timing of metastatic disease, it does, of course, depend greatly on how advanced the cancer was initially. Statistically, metastatic disease can occur as early as one year after an initial diagnosis of breast cancer to as late as forty years after initial treatment.

SYMPTOMS OF A SPREAD

As discussed earlier in this chapter, if you have been treated for a life-threatening illness, you may wish to consider keeping a health diary to record how you are feeling on a daily or weekly basis. That way, if you do experience suspicious symptoms (which may or may not indicate metastatic disease), it may be easier to report them to your doctors. However, it's also important to keep in mind that just because you had—or have—breast cancer, it doesn't mean you can't get sick with the garden variety aches and pains (colds, flus, etc.) like the rest of the population.

While most of the ailments cancer patients suffer from are not due to cancer, some symptoms to watch for:

1. *Dry, persistent cough.* This indicates a problem with the lungs.
2. *Difficulty breathing or shortness of breath.* Again, this indicates a problem with the lungs.

3. *General aches and pains or stiffness.* This can indicate that the cancer has spread to the bones.

4. *Enlarged lymph nodes—anywhere.* Lymph nodes under the arms, neck, collar bone area, and groin area should be checked regularly. Immediately report any enlargement to your doctor.

5. *General fatigue.* This is a sign that you are fighting off something. It could be the flu; it could be cancer. Report this to your doctor.

6. *Sores that don't heal, or rashes, especially in the upper body.* Breast cancer can recur on the surface of the skin. Get it looked at immediately.

7. *Changes in weight or appetite and/or fevers.* This is a sign of a possible problem in the liver.

8. *Headaches and/or vision problems that get progressively worse with time.* These are signs of cancer in the brain or eye region. However, a headache can just mean a headache! (Brain metastasis occurs in only about 6 percent of women with breast cancer.)

9. *Muscle weakness or paralysis.* This can be a sign of brain or spinal cord metastasis.

10. *Extreme, localized pain along your spinal column.* This is a sign of metastasis to the spinal cord—not a common site, however.

WHAT DID I DO TO CAUSE THIS?

Nothing. Many women look back at their first set of treatment decisions and wonder if they made the right choices. For instance, if you decided initially not to have chemotherapy and are now facing metastatic disease, could you have prevented it by adjuvant therapy? Or, if you had a wide excision or partial mastectomy versus a modified radical mastectomy, or no hormone therapy, and so on, could this have been prevented? Nobody knows the answers to these questions, but what I can tell you is that plenty of women who did all the "right things" the first time around (modified radical mastectomies, followed by adjuvant chemotherapy) face metastatic disease, too.

The only question to ask is this: did I make the initial treatment decisions to the best of my ability at the time? And most of us do. This time around, you can only do the same.

TREATING METASTATIC DISEASE

Once breast cancer advances to this stage, there is no one way to treat the disease. Here are just a few of the factors taken into consideration when deciding treatment:

1. *How much time has passed since the initial cancer was diagnosed?* The more time that's passed, the better the prognosis.

2. *Is this breast cancer well-differentiated or poorly differentiated?* The better differentiated, the better the prognosis. (See Chapter 3 for more information.)

3. *Is the cancer estrogen-receptor positive? If it is, is it easier to treat?* (See Chapter 4 for more information.)

4. *How many places has the cancer spread?* Obviously, the less, the better.

5. *Which sites have breast cancer?* Breast cancer multiplies faster in certain parts of the body, such as the liver, slower in bone.

6. *How severe are the symptoms?* If you can barely breath, radiation therapy may be used to shrink the size of the tumor for optimal comfort. A lack of symptoms may warrant a different approach.

7. *What is the age of the patient?* Chemotherapy may be too harsh if you are elderly and too frail to tolerate the side effects.

Other factors to consider are the goals of the treatment and the extent to which you want treatment. Many women with metastatic breast cancer choose alternative therapies over more aggressive Western therapies. Many women opt for palliative care in conjunction with alternative healing. (Palliative care is discussed in the next chapter.)

So, treatment will vary, depending on the desired outcome: cure or prolonging survival (if a cure isn't possible) or relief of symptoms or maintaining quality of life for as along as possible (that is, postponing treatment for as long as possible).

Support groups and friendship in general have been shown to prolong survival in women with metastatic disease. One well-respected 1989 study showed that women with metastatic disease who had a weekly support group added to their usual care as well as other friendships lived eighteen months longer than those with no support.

Options on the table

If you have no symptoms, you may decide to carry on as before and live life to the fullest. After all, having cancer doesn't mean you're suddenly mortal; it simply means you are facing mortality sooner than the woman who gets killed suddenly in a car accident. No treatment is certainly a worthwhile consideration when the side effects of treatment are worse than the disease itself.

Obviously, if a cure is entirely possible, you'll probably want to go for it. This can involve radiation (used in these cases to shrink tumors), sometimes followed by surgery (where operable), chemotherapy, and hormone therapy (see further on).

Researchers at Duke University found that women with metastatic disease were better off waiting until they had a recurrence before they went onto chemotherapy and bone marrow transplants. Women who waited until the recurrence seemed to have less side-effects from the therapy and seemed to have improved survival rates.

Hormone therapy

Although discussed in detail in Chapter 4, it's important to note here that hormone therapy is often the recommended treatment for women with metastatic disease. Hormone therapy in reproductive cancers is an area that is seeing the most progress in terms of drug development; it is reserved for cancers that are not growing rapidly in vital organs.

In premenopausal women, the goal of hormone therapy is to stop the ovaries from producing estrogen. When tamoxifen is not used, the ovaries can be radiated or surgically removed. See pages 148–149 for details.

Chemotherapy

When cancer is growing rapidly, or is not responding to hormone therapy, chemotherapy is often considered. The combination of drugs in this case depends on what you had the first time around. Usually, if you had adjuvant chemotherapy at least a year before your recurrence, the same drugs that were used before are administered in a different combination of dosages. If your adjuvant chemotherapy was administered less than a year ago, usually the drug Taxol, or Paclitaxel, is used. This drug can have disturbing side effects that include flushing, shortness of breath, skin rashes, decrease of white blood cells, diarrhea, nausea, vomiting, numbness, and joint pains.

In this case, chemotherapy is given for as long as it can be, as long as you're responding. Often, the side effects of metastatic disease can be alleviated through chemotherapy—side effects such as shortness of breath (if cancer is in the lungs), bone aches, and tumors of the skin or liver or abdomen. What chemotherapy will not be able to do is to take away the fatigue that metastatic disease usually causes.

Radiation

In metastatic disease, radiation therapy is often used as a symptom-reliever. Because it can shrink tumors, radiation can relieve the pressure in a number of areas, and thus your pain. Radiation is often given at the same time as hormone therapy or chemotherapy. If your cancer has spread to the bone, radiation is particularly helpful because it will shrink the tumor and relieve the pressure in the bone, preventing further bone damage.

You will feel relief usually within a month. Radiation is more effective for bone pain also because the bone can tolerate far higher doses of radiation than other parts of the body and because pain is often effectively relieved by radiation. Bones, unlike many parts of the body, can be treated with radiation more than once.

When cancer is in the chest wall, radiation can sometimes shrink the tumor to make it operable, or it can relieve the pressure on the lungs. When the cancer has spread to the skin, radiation can be used repeatedly if necessary..

When the cancer has spread to the brain, radiation is sometimes the only form of therapy that can be used; although chemotherapy is sometimes effective as well. Fatigue, nausea, headaches, and hair loss are the most common symptoms of radiation to the head.

When is surgery used?

When breast cancer has spread to the bones, surgery can be used to avoid fractures or to mend already fractured bone. In this case, an orthopedic surgeon is called in.

Surgery is sometimes used to remove individual tumors on the skin and in the lungs, liver, or even brain.

FLUID ACCUMULATION

This is a condition that often occurs when cancer spreads to the lungs and blocks the lymph nodes that drain the area. Fluid begins to accumulate, causing shortness of breath and sharp chest pain, especially when taking breaths.

If you have these symptoms, a physical exam and chest X ray will confirm the diagnosis. Treatment consists of draining the fluid by inserting a tube into the chest. Antibiotics are also used to help fight off infection in the area.

Sometimes fluid can accumulate in the abdomen, causing swelling and bloating. An ultrasound and a physical exam will confirm the problem. A catheter is inserted into the abdomen to drain the fluid.

• • • • • • •

The next chapter discusses an important aspect of cancer therapy: palliative care. Many think of palliative care as a step reserved for advanced disease, but this is not so. Palliative care is about quality of life at any stage of an illness.

CHAPTER 9

PALLIATIVE CARE

Palliative care refers to symptom relief and is a component of all medical care, whether the intent is to cure a disease or to eliminate its symptoms. People will want to be free of spiritual, psychological, and physical symptoms at all stages of an illness, from the earliest stage of diagnosis until they are cured, or die. But what does it mean to treat the symptoms of a disease, rather than the disease itself? Sometimes all it boils down to is different goals. For example, palliative care is often the exact opposite of chemotherapy, which may cause more symptoms than the cancer itself.

When it comes to breast cancer, palliative care is an option that more and more women with metastatic disease are choosing because it promotes quality of life and allows one to enjoy the time one has left. And, after the soul-searching they go through, many cancer patients will tell you that, in the final analysis, that's what life's all about anyway.

Now, palliative care and all the various forms of treatment discussed in this book (such as radiation, chemotherapy, surgery, complementary medicine, and so on) are not mutually exclusive. Many of these therapies can treat symptoms, and thus fall into the broad category of palliative care.

To a Western medical practitioner, palliative medicine is about pain and symptom management. So, yes, we are talking about the use of powerful narcotics in a lot of cases. In a healthy person, narcotic drugs are addictive and dull abilities and life functions. But when administered for palliative care, narcotics dull the pain, enabling the person to function normally. And when narcotics are administered by a trained specialist, addiction simply isn't a concern. I'll go into this issue in more detail beginning on page 244.

TREATING THE SYMPTOMS: PALLIATIVE CARE

Whenever medicine or therapy is needed to relieve the pain or symptoms of an illness, this is known as "palliative care." Palliative care generally enters into the breast cancer picture when metastatic disease has developed and there are no therapies available that can cure the disease. In this case, the goals of therapy change from what doctors call a curative approach, meaning that therapies and medications are designed to cure the cancer, to a palliative approach, where medications and therapies are designed not to cure, but to make patients comfortable and alert so that they can carry on as normally as possible.

WHO IS A PALLIATIVE CARE PATIENT?

Anyone who wants to be free of the symptoms of her disease is a palliative care patient. In other words, you don't have to have a time limit placed on your life before you can receive palliative care. Many women with breast cancer live for several years as palliative care patients and are able to have a good quality of life. In fact, you can request a palliative approach at any time during your treatment. The request will be followed by consultations with your oncologists, who will refer you to a palliative care team at your medical center. The palliative care team may consist of a palliative care physician, as well as your family and friends for support. Or, a larger team may be brought in that consists of several consulting doctors, nurses, a physiotherapist, a pharmacist, a psychologist, a social worker, clergy, a dietitian, and volunteers.

Palliative care is also "portable." Depending on your health, you can receive treatment as an outpatient through regular visits to the hospital or to the palliative care specialist, or you may be hospitalized.

How you should be treated

You have the right to expect the following from your palliative care team:

1. *An open-ended approach to therapy.* In other words, your care should be flexible to meet your changing needs, rather than rigid and finite.
2. *No blanket reassurances that everything will be fine.* Your team should be frank about your prognosis but sensitive to your feelings.
3. *As much information as you want, whenever you want it.*
4. *Jargon-free explanations.* This means non-technical descriptions of what's happening in your body and non-technical descriptions of the therapy recommended to relieve symptoms.
5. *Ongoing assessment.* You should be regularly assessed by your doctor and informed about your illness's progression and what symptoms to expect. Your health may be changing daily.
6. *Participation in your treatment.*
7. *The goals of your treatment defined in black and white.* For example, if you're having radiation therapy to your chest area to shrink a tumor, the goal is to shrink the tumor so you can breathe more easily—not to cure the cancer.
8. *Techniques for coping with family and friends.* You should be able to count on your team for supportive advice in dealing with family or friends who are in conflict or denial about your situation.

THE SYMPTOMS

One of the most common symptoms of advanced cancer is shortness of breath. This can be caused by a number of factors such as fluid accumulation, pneumonia, hyperventiliation, and a tumor pressing down on the lungs. All these conditions can be treated: fluid accumulation can be removed; pneumonia can be treated with antibiotics; hyperventillation due to anxiety can be relieved through breathing techniques or anti-anxiety medications; a tumor pressing down on the lungs may require you to be on oxygen at home or in the hospital.

If there is no way to remove the cause of shortness of breath, narcotics such as morphine and hydromorphine will decrease the sensation of breathlessness.

Loss of appetite (called anorexia) is another common symptom associated with advanced cancer. Sometimes appetite loss has to do with where your cancer is located; other times it is a response to pain medication. The most upsetting aspect of appetite loss is what it does to the people around you. So the first rule is to have your palliative team reassure your family and friends that food is not a guarantee of a longer life span. Generally, dietitians recommend that you have people prepare foods in very small portions, in the "single-wrapped" or "finger food" formats. You'll find food much more appetizing this way. Meal replacement drinks, which have a fair bit of calories and vitamins, can also solve some problems. You can sip from a can or two throughout the day.

Mild to severe nausea is also a symptom in advanced cancer and is caused either by the new location to which your cancer has spread or due to various medications. The solutions vary from anti-nausea medications to adjusting diet or medications.

You may also have constipattion, a classic symptom of narcotic pain relief, which can be alleviated with laxatives and stool softeners.

Bladder incontinence can be another symptom. It is alleviated with either a catheter or bladder control undergarments.

Fatigue strikes again with advanced cancer. Fatigue at this time is often a sign that you are not sleeping well at night because your pain wakes you up. This means that you need a stronger pain-control medication, discussed further on. Fatigue can, of course, be a side effect of treatments such as radiation or of narcotic medications such as codeine and morphine.

WHEN PAIN HURTS

You can be seriously ill and have no severe physical pain and require nothing more than some over-the-counter drugs. But when advanced cancer causes severe pain, you're going to need some strong stuff to control it. Your doctor will usually start with a non-narcotic and work up to a narcotic painkiller, known as an opioid (the root word is *opium,* one of the oldest narcotics). Narcotic medication for severe pain control is generally not addictive in the sense that you don't wait for your next "fix," nor do you become "strung out" on drugs. Many narcotics also come in pain patches (worn on the skin like nicotine patches), which eliminate much of the dosage administering of days gone by.

But when the drug wears off, you will feel the pain again; so you'll want another dose just to feel *normal*. And that's fine—that's what a narcotic is designed to do.

While narcotics may be a godsend, they are still, of course, powerful drugs. You can't just take them by yourself when you feel like it. You're going to need someone who is an expert at administering the lowest possible dose of a narcotic. The dose is based on a number of factors: where your pain is located; the cause of your pain; how much pain you have; and your overall health. But patients and their families are now being encouraged by specialists to become their own experts in managing and administering their narcotic dosages.

WHY ALL THE PAIN?

Pain is a sign that something is wrong. You already know that now, but your body doesn't *know* you do. In the same way that a smoke detector will continue to ring until the smoke clears, your body will continue to send pain signals until you remove the cause of the pain. Until that day comes (which is probably unlikely in advanced cancer), you have to deaden the pain. Your nerve endings act as the "smoke detectors" in your body. Every part of your body has free nerve endings, while the spinal cord has pain receptors that receive the pain sent by the nerve endings.

Sometimes it's the nerves themselves that are damaged, due to nerve compression or spinal cord compression. This causes that intermittent, stabbing pain, often accompanied by a burning sensation or numbness. Pain can also be caused by tumors that infiltrate bone or press down on other organs. This will lead to more continuous, aching pains.

Pain has many shapes and forms, which help tell your palliative care team what's going on. For example, acute pain has a clear beginning, middle, and end, as well as physical signs such as sweating, pupil dilation, and a pounding heart.

Chronic pain is harder to describe because it goes on and on in a continuous aching. It's sometimes difficult for your doctors to tell if you have chronic pain because people tend to describe it as discomfort or "unwellness." In some, chronic pain triggers depression, irritability, or sleeplessness. Or, as the illness advances and you become more debilitated, depressed, or anxious, your awareness of pain increases; this makes the pain feel worse (even though it may actually be the same pain you've been dealing with for a while).

There is another condition known as total pain, when you're just "maxed out" from a variety of pains related to your illness: pain from the disease itself; pain as a side effect of treatment or medication; emotional pain, and so on.

PAIN MANAGEMENT

The number one goal of pain management in cancer is to prevent or completely control pain. Period. No exceptions. So the first thing your doctor will do is to try and figure out what's causing your pain. For example, if a tumor is pressing down on an organ, it can often be shrunk with radiation, or surgically removed, thus eliminating the pain without resorting to narcotic drugs.

Your doctor will also try to get you to assess your pain on a number system from 0 to 5, where 0 = no pain; 1 = mild pain; 2 = discomforting pain; 3 = distressing pain; 4 = horrible pain; and 5 = excruciating pain. This will tell your doctor what type of medications you need for pain control. Obviously, a 5 will require the "hard stuff," while a 2 or 3 may be managed with a non-narcotic medication.

Drugs that control pain

There are classes of drugs used to control pain that doctors prescribe in a stepped-care approach. That means they start with the least powerful drug and work their way up as the pain increases.

On the bottom step is a class of drugs known as non-opioids (a.k.a. non-narcotics). These are basic pain killers (analgesics) such as acetylsalicylic acid or A.S.A.(aspirin) and acetaminophen (Tylenol) and non-steroidal anti-inflammatory drugs (NSAIDs) such as ibuprofen or naproxen (Naprosyn). These drugs work by interfering with body chemicals called *prostaglandins*, which normally cause inflammation and increase your body's pain receptor "firing." Non-narcotics are used not just for mild pain, but for bone pain and other forms of severe pain.

The second step up the pain ladder is what's called a weak opioid, which is often mixed with a non-opioid. Codeine is a weak opioid, and it's often mixed with acetaminophen in a drug such as Tylenol 3.

The third and final step up is a strong opioid such as morphine or hydromorphone. Both strong and weak opioids are known as narcotics. They work in the central nervous system (the brain and spinal cord), inhibiting the transmission of pain. Narcotics commonly used in advanced cancer treatment are morphine preparations and hydromorphine (Dilaudid). Less common are propoxyphene (Darvon), oxycodone (Percodan), and oxymorphone (Numorphan).

Co-analgesics

On any step in the pain management ladder, your doctor may decide to combine the analgesic with a drug that will relieve other symptoms of your illness, or prevent the side effects of your painkiller. For example, anticonvulsants, antidepressants, steroids, membrane stabilizing drugs, or anti-anxiety drugs may all be added to non-opioids, weak opioids, or strong opioids.

Taking drugs as needed versus round-the-clock drugs

As discussed earlier, depending on the kind of pain you have, your doctor will want to prevent it or control it. To prevent pain, you'll be on what's called a "regular" dosing schedule whether you have pain or not. This is better than "waiting" for the pain to build up and much less stressful for you. In this case, however, you must take the dose as prescribed—no more drug, no less drug taken no more frequently or less frequently. Otherwise, either the pain will not be managed properly or else too much of the drug will build up in your system so that it becomes toxic to your general health.

Taking medications as needed (known as p.r.n. in pharmacyspeak) is a little trickier. You must take the drug as soon as you start to feel the least bit uncomfortable. If you wait until the pain increases (to "tough it out" until it gets really bad), the drug just won't work as well, and you'll have to take higher doses. Of course, it may well be that you do not need to be on as high a dose of the drug as you are or that another drug may work better. So be on the lookout for post-dose symptoms such as agitation, or extreme drowsiness after taking a drug—it may mean that your doctor needs to adjust the dosage or change the drug.

ISSUES SURROUNDING NARCOTICS

So long as your doctor knows what's causing your pain, you should be able to have as many analgesics as you need to control the pain. In fact, nurses on palliative care wards in hospitals should have standing orders to increase the pain medication if it's not strong enough.

Dosing is another issue around narcotics. There is no standard or maximum dose for these medications. Dosing varies with the individual situation and the individual. So it's important for you or your family (if you are not able) to keep a diary of when you're experiencing pain so you and your doctor can develop a regular dosing schedule that prevents what's called breakthrough pain.

Balancing your medications is another issue, particularly when co-analgesics (see preceding section) are added to your pain medications. Ask your doctor or pharmacist to draw up a chart that you can follow that lists all the medications you need to take and when you need to take them. It's usually fine to take all your various medications as a group (analgesic, anti-depressant, and narcotic) in the morning, for example, and at other times in the day as prescribed. This is easier than taking, say, your analgesic at 8:00 A.M., your anti-depressant at 10:00 A.M. and your narcotic at noon, and then repeating this a second or third time. It would be enough to confuse anybody!

Constipation, discussed briefly earlier, is a major side effect of narcotics and is aggravated by a lower fluid and food intake and less mobility. Laxatives and stool softeners should be combined with any narcotic medication you're on. In fact, herbal laxatives may work beautifully in this situation (see Chapter 7).

IF YOU'RE NOT FINDING RELIEF

Most people do best with a combination of prescription and over-the-counter painkillers. Specialists usually encourage their patients to manage painkillers on their own as much as possible. Since you are, after all, the one experiencing your pain, it's presumed that you would be more knowledgeable on your pain than anyone else. If you are not finding relief, however, there may be some inappropriate administration behind this, rather than a narcotic drug that is "not working." Is the doctor prescribing the drug regularly, around the clock? Is the drug's duration of action matched to its dosing schedule? In other words, if the drug's effect lasts for two hours, but it is only being prescribed every four, you'll be in pain for two hours in between! That's not a proper way for a painkiller to be administered. It is possible that you are not finding relief simply because you need a stronger dose of the drug.

Ironically, the longer you're made to wait for the next dose of the drug, the more pain you will feel due to anticipation and stress. Worse, you're more likely to get dependent on a drug and "clock watch," when you're forced to wait for relief.

WHAT YOU SHOULDN'T WORRY ABOUT

A common concern for palliative care patients is that large doses of narcotics will mean even larger doses in the future. This isn't true. Once your doctor finds the right dose to successfully manage your pain (which can take a few tries), you shouldn't need a dose increase unless your pain increases—which will happen not because you've become too used to the narcotic, but because your disease is progressing. If your dosage is not sufficiently controlling your pain, you must discuss this with your physician and ask for a pain assessment.

Dependence or addiction is another common fear, but it really shouldn't be a concern if the drug is being administered appropriately.

THE PROBLEM YOU DON'T READ ABOUT

More and more cancer patients these days are selling their narcotic prescriptions to drug abusers on the street. These prescriptions can be worth hundreds or even thousands of dollars, which makes selling drugs tempting. Doctors are beginning to catch on to this phenomenon and become suspicious if patients claim that their prescription was stolen, outdated, or borrowed by a friend or family member.

Doctors are currently managing this problem by prescribing narcotics that are not "pure." That is, the drugs are a mixture of analgesics, co-analgesics, and the narcotic. If the motivation to sell your prescription is profit, because you can't afford to pay for your treatment, speak to your practitioners about financing before you resort to this. The last thing you need is to be arrested (which will happen if you're caught).

ISSUES SURROUNDING END-STAGE CANCER

If you're in poor health, at some point you'll need to decide whether you want to be treated at home, in a hospital, or somewhere in between such as a hospice. What factors into the decision is the availability of homecare or a caregiver, equipment such as an adjustable bed, bedside pans, IV lines, comfort devices such as special mattresses, hand rails, mechanical aids for the bath/shower, oxygen and suction equipment, walkers, chairs, wheelchairs, and so on. If you're currently hospitalized, you can request an overnight pass and try going home for a night to see whether your family is able to give you the kind of care you require. This is one way to experiment with different arrangements.

Sometimes the solution is to go in for respite care, meaning temporary hospital stays that give your family or a paid caregiver some time off from caregiving. Temporary hospital stays can last from one to two weeks.

More and more hospitals are encouraging patients to receive palliative care at home, due to rising costs or a decrease in the number of beds available. At any rate, it is important to make sure that you're in an environment with:

1. Proper equipment and resources.
2. Access to ongoing assessment.

3. Access to proper symptom and pain control.

4. Access to caregiver substitutes to relieve caregiver exhaustion.

5. Access to emergency care in the case of a problem.

"BUT IT'S NOT LIKE ME TO BEHAVE THIS WAY"

If you're dealing with end-stage cancer, don't be ashamed or surprised if you suddenly start behaving differently. Your palliative care team, family, and friends already know this isn't "like you." So there's no need to feel guilty or to apologize for yourself. The most common behaviors are yelling at people for no reason and blaming people for your predicament. This happens when you're so angry about your illness that you don't know what to do. So things get a little out of control. Big deal. Just recognize what's happening and try to focus your anger on the right "subject"—your cancer. You're angry at the cancer, not at your loved ones.

Some women become aware that they get "chatty" when their practitioners come by, and may notice a change in their practitioner's manner. This chattiness comes from feelings of anxiety and sometimes of isolation. Counseling or support groups will help to relieve these feelings.

DEALING WITH OPEN TUMORS ON THE SKIN

This is not an uncommon condition. Sometimes tumors can erode through the skin and behave like a large open wound. This can create some trauma for you or your family if you're not prepared, because, like any open wound, an open tumor can have an unpleasant odor and attract anaerobic organisms. In the same way that you can't smell your own breath, you may not notice an odor even if it exists. In some cases, patients may wish (or need) to be moved to a private room. Radiation therapy is usually the first step in treating this condition; it will often resolve the problem. Otherwise, the tumor must be dressed and cleaned once or twice daily (rarely more often than that) to avoid further trauma or cauterized if bleeding is a problem. If you should find yourself with an open tumor, it is important to ask your palliative care team for a detailed briefing about the symptoms you should expect and the appropriate way to care for the wound. In most cases such wounds are painless, and the odor can be eliminated by treating the anaerobic infection with topical metronidazole.

· · · · · · ·

The final chapter in this book answers the question: What can my daughter do to prevent this from happening to her? There are many theories about breast cancer prevention, (which I discuss), but there is little consensus about really concrete prevention strategies. As a result, many angry and frustrated breast cancer survivors and family members are taking their feelings to the grassroots level of the problem. In the last five years, hundreds of patient-led support groups, information vehicles, and organizations have started up to help give breast cancer a more prevention-led focus and future.

CHAPTER 10

WHAT ABOUT PREVENTION?

There's a world of difference between the terms *prevention* and *detection*. There is also a vast difference between primary prevention and secondary prevention. Right now, when the medical community discusses "preventing breast cancer" it means detecting breast cancer. Breast self exam and breast screening via mammography is detection, NOT prevention. Some will call BSE and mammography secondary prevention. But primary prevention means changing the behavior that causes the disease.

Many diseases, such as AIDS, can be prevented. And some cancers, such as cervical cancer or skin cancer, can be prevented. But breast cancer is not the kind of cancer that can be prevented since we don't really know what causes it to begin with.

For example, if environmental toxins are responsible for a large majority of breast cancer, primary prevention means eliminating these toxins from the environment. Lobbying for environmental protection laws is therefore one way you can help to prevent breast cancer. If our dietary fat serves as a host for these toxins, then changing our diet is a form of primary prevention. And finally, since we know for sure that women who breastfeed as long as possible develop less breast cancer, then breastfeeding or supporting other women to breastfeed (like your daughters or granddaughters), is an active form of primary prevention.

In the first chapter of this book, we looked at the myriad of conflicting studies regarding breast cancer risk. And we discovered that there are no sure-fire answers. Well it's the same with the area of breast cancer prevention. There is no magic food, magic herb, or magic exercise that can prevent breast cancer. In fact, one medical advisor for this book told me flat out that it was "cruel" to present information about breast cancer prevention in absolute terms, such as "You can prevent breast cancer by cutting your dietary fat." Unfortunately, it's easy to find articles and books that contain those kinds of prescriptions, and there are plenty of women out there who did exactly what they prescribed—ate broccoli, stopped eating meat, and so on—and still developed breast cancer. Nevertheless, there are many things you can do to become healthier and stronger today. There are also ways to improve the information and education about breast cancer, nutrition, and general health that we give to the next generation so that detection can take place earlier and earlier. The central message of this chapter is this: The most we can do to be healthy right now is the best we can do.

So while this chapter discusses how to effect dietary changes that can make a difference in your overall health, it is not a prescription for breast cancer prevention.

This chapter also discusses some prevention strategies employed by the medical community, such as the controversial health trial with the drug tamoxifen. It also discusses prevention surgery, something that women are looking into more and more.

Finally, this chapter addresses breast cancer education and activism. The more information our daughters and granddaughters have about this disease, the more proactive they can become about breast cancer detection, treatment, diagnosis, and, one day, perhaps prevention.

THE ROLE OF DIET

The word *diet* comes from the Greek word *diatta,* which means way of life. Of course, in more modern times, the word *diet* has come to be associated with a narrower definition—weight loss or a restricted diet regimen. The term *diatta* obviously has much broader implications.

To a large extent, many of us *are* eating the wrong things and eating too much. We have been doing so especially since the Industrial Revolution brought about widespread changes in food technology. We began to see more modern diseases, such as tuberculosis, stomach ailments, and cancers, around this time, as well. In fact, these diseases are linked by many nutritionists to the invention of refined flour and the changes in water supply.

We also know that breast cancer rates are four to seven times higher in the United States than they are in Asia, but that genetics seem to have little to do with this. When Asian women move to the United States, their risk doubles over a decade, and they seem to acquire breast cancer at United States rates after several generations. We just don't know what accounts for this difference. Is it diet? Are we eating something we shouldn't, or are they eating some foods that we should? Or, do they stop eating certain foods when they emigrate to the West? For example, the average Japanese diet has roughly 15 percent of its calories from fat; the American diet gets 40 percent of its calories from fat. The traditional Japanese diet of rice, vegetables, and fish is eons away from the meat and fat of North American diets. But the Japanese diet is also rich in plant estrogens (called photoestrogens or phytoestrogens) such as tofu. Photoestrogens act as weak estrogens, and weak estrogens interfere with ordinary estrogen production. If estrogen promotes breast tumors, then anything that interferes with estrogen production should theoretically cut the risk. Some studies suggest that this is so: photoestrogens may be associated with lower rates of breast cancer and less severe menopausal symptoms. Photoestrogens can be found in a variety of fruits and vegetables, including all soybean and linseed products, apples, alfalfa sprouts, split peas, and spinach.

Perhaps culture is a large piece in the puzzle. People in Western cultures have fewer children, more birth control, and less breastfeeding, while Asian cultures favor more children, more breastfeeding, and less birth control. Some even wonder whether the more physical lifestyle of Asian women versus the sedentary lifestyle of Western women can play a role.

No matter what the reasons are for this statistical difference in breast cancer rates between East and West, *everyone* agrees that the Western diet contains more calories, more fat, and more meat than other diets, which absolutely leads to heart disease and strokes—diseases that kill more women than breast cancer. How did the Western diet get so unhealthy, anyway? Well, technology has a lot to do with it.

REFINED DIETS

The early twentieth century saw the rise of the petrochemical industry in the United States and Western Europe, which coincided with the rise of more advanced surgery and pharmacological approaches. The growth of the petrochemical industry led to chemical agriculture and factory farming, which revolutionized food consumption patterns. In fact, this development created a huge oxymoron: As we became more modern in food distribution, nutrition knowledge suffered. This is evident in the fact that modern medical schools generally devote very little time to nutrition in their curriculum.

Meanwhile, back in the kitchen, general nutritional neglect became widespread. And as our diet began to include high fat, refined carbohydrates, chemical additives, and other nutritional variables, cancer rates began to rise as well. Epidemiologists already know that cultures that stick to a traditional diet of whole grains, cooked vegetables, and fresh seasonal fruit have fewer cases, cancer. But, as discussed in Chapter 1, there may be other factors at work here: longevity rates, differences in family sizes, and a host of other factors that diet studies may not be looking at.

A QUESTION OF OVERNUTRITION

Hippocrates referred to cancer as a disease of "overnutrition" (when you look at today's statistics, you know he may have been onto something). The "refined" things in life such as sugar, white flour, and other refined foods—coupled with excess protein and fat—contribute to a number of diseases. For proof, just do a tour of duty through a pharmacy shelf and look at the number of antacids and constipation remedies available.

Many Eastern nutritionists see the Western diet as the cause of world poverty and hunger. Modern agricultural systems use the majority of arable land for livestock production and cash crops such as tomatoes, sugar, coffee, and bananas. Currently, 80 percent of our grain harvest goes to feed cattle for milk and slaughter and to feed other livestock. But in the Third World, tens of millions of families growing grains and vegetables have been uprooted by cattle and sugar plantations. The result is that these families get crowded into cities, which forms slums, which leads to the downward spiral we're so familiar with: hunger, disease, and crime.

For thousands of years, cooked whole grains were a dietary staple. In the Orient it was rice and millet; in Europe, wheat, oats, and rye; in Russia and Communist Asia, buckwheat; in Africa, sorghum; barley in the Middle East; and corn in the Americas.

Of course, you couldn't find a diet in the West that is based on grains. We consume, by any standards, an obscene amount of meat. The proof is in the statistics put out by the United States Department of Agriculture (USDA). Between 1910 and 1976, wheat consumption dropped by 48 percent, corn by 85 percent, rye by 78 percent, barley by 66 percent, buckwheat by 98 percent, beans and legumes by 46 percent, fresh vegetables by 23 percent, and fresh fruit by 33 percent.

Meanwhile, the consumption of beef rose by 72 percent, poultry by 194 percent, cheese by 322 percent, canned vegetables by 320 percent, frozen vegetables by 1,650 percent, processed fruit by 556 percent, and soft drinks by 2,638 percent. And since 1940, chemical additives and preservatives in our food have risen by 995 percent.

Theoretically, excessive eating interferes with our body's ability to discharge toxins. Some theorize that when layers of fat develop under the skin, this could lead to deposits of mucous and fat, which may also affect the breasts.

The meat of the issue

In its report on the impact of modern farming and food processing, the American Association of Advancement of Science stated that a diet centered on whole-grain cereals and vegetables rather than meat and poultry would benefit our entire way of life, making more land, water, fuel, and minerals available, which would in turn have positive effects on inflation, employment, and international trade.

In 1991, researchers at the California Institute of Technology reported that a meat-based diet was actually ruining the environment. Apparently, cooking meat contributes to air pollution because it releases hydrocarbons, furans, steroids, and pesticide residues. Interestingly, a major source of smog in Los Angeles is smoke from *barbecued beef!* In light of this, I think it's time for carnivores like me to really review our diets and make some thoughtful changes. It may just happen.

On Earth Day 1992 an international coalition of environmental groups pledged to help lower beef consumption by 50 percent by the year 2002. The plan is to move toward a diet centered around whole grains and vegetables. In fact, there may even come a day when meat and high-fat foods are heavily taxed (a "sin tax") to remind us that we are what we eat.

FAT STUDIES STILL THIN

As of this writing, studies on dietary fat and breast cancer have not been able to prove that high-fat diets are linked to a greater breast cancer risk. BUT—studies suggest that a low-fat diet may make breast cancers easier to detect because they can reduce the density of your breast tissue. After two years, study participants on a low-fat, high-carbohydrate diet were able to reduce the area of density on a mammogram, making the mammogram more accurate. Environmental scientists such as Dr. Sandra Steingraber, in her book *Living Downstream,* also point out that fat is a host for environmental toxins. The more fat on your body, the more inviting you make it for *uninvited* toxins. Italian studies showed that breast cancer risk was associated with diets high in: saturated fat (greatest risk), alcohol (lesser risk), and starch (least risk of the three). The fat-and-breast-cancer issue has certainly polarized breast cancer researchers. Many will tell you the proof is in the geography: countries with high-fat diets simply have more breast cancer. Others will tell you that there are too many geographical and cultural variables that need to be studied before the fat theory becomes fact.

You've probably heard about the Nurses' Health study, in which half the nurses enrolled got 44 percent of their daily calories from fat, while the other half got 23 percent of their daily calories from fat. The nurses were followed over several years. Harvard University's Walter Willett recently analyzed the results. He concluded that the study showed *no* difference in breast cancer risk between the two groups. Similar studies on dietary fat have found the same results.

Critics of the Nurses' Health Study argue that in order to prove a difference, the "fat-cutting nurses" should have been getting no more than 15 percent of their calories from fat. Other studies have other problems. Many use food frequency questionnaires to measure what people are eating, and these questionnaires are a pretty crude measurement tool. Researchers have also raised the issue of the "timing" of dietary fat in a woman's life cycle. Some wonder whether low-fat diets have a greater impact on breast cancer risk when taken in childhood and adolescence, when breasts are still forming, than in adulthood.

We may know the answers to some of these questions in the year 2010, when the results from the largest dietary fat study to date are due. The Women's Health Initiative (which breast cancer activists point out should have started several years ago) is a $628 million health trial involving 164,000 women. It intends to test whether a low-fat diet that is high in fruits, vegetables, and grains leads to lower breast cancer incidence in postmenopausal women than the typical Western diet. If you're interested in participating, are healthy, and past menopause, you can call the Women's Health Initiative directly at 1-800-54-WOMEN.

MAKING CHANGES

It is only natural that you want to eat well to be as healthy as you can possibly be today. For the majority of us, that means making some changes in our diet. We do know that women who eat low-fat diets and who exercise have much lower rates of heart disease and stroke.

Eating well essentially means eating less fat, more fruits, all colors of vegetables, and lots of whole grains for fiber.

GOOD FATS/BAD FATS

Fat is by far the most damaging element in the Western diet. This fat comes from meats, dairy products, and vegetable oils. Other sources of fat include coconuts (60 percent fat), peanuts (78 percent fat), and avocadoes (82 percent fat). The latest theory is that diets with only 20 percent of calories from fat will probably serve you well. But it is hard to tell the good fats from the bad fats in your diet. There is a difference.

Olive oil, for example, is a good fat. It is a monounsaturated fat that tends to decrease the low density lipids (LDL) in your bloodstream. LDL is also known as "bad" cholesterol. When LDL decreases, the "good" cholesterol, high density lipids (HDL), increases. Olive oil's goodness has been shown in studies that looked at breast cancer in Greek, southern Italian, and Spanish women. Although the large proportion of olive oil in their diets didn't affect their breast cancer rates, it has been suggested that olive oil is a "good" oil. We still don't know for sure if olive oil actually protects against breast cancer, or simply replaces more dangerous fats in the diets. Animals fed olive oil in laboratory tests had fewer breast tumors than animals that were fed safflower or corn oil.

Omega-3 oils, which are found mainly in fatty fish, and which have been proven to be beneficial to the heart, may also have a protective effect against tumors. Fish that contain these oils are salmon (natural only, not "farm-raised"), mackerel, sable, whitefish, herring, and sardines. Apparently, you must eat these fish frequently in order to derive any protection.

High quality sesame oil and corn oil are also considered better oils to cook with. Sesame oil is found in Japanese diets.

Solid evidence

The best way to determine what fat is bad is to see how solid it is at room temperature. So, things like lard, butter, margarine, and solid vegetable shortening, for example, are very bad fats. They're high in saturated fat and should be avoided. In fact, the way the fat looks just before you eat it is the way it will look when it lines your arteries. So, if you're lured into the low-calorie world of margarine and solid vegetable shortening, don't be fooled: They're no better than plain butter or lard because they contain trans-fatty acids, which have been linked to cardiovascular disease. Trans-fatty acids are made from a process called hydrogenation (which solidifies oils).

Saturated fat

Okay, ladies—here's the definition of saturated fats: anything that stimulates your body to make cholesterol is a saturated fat. In other words, a saturated fat is a cholesterol stimulant and is worse than foods that are naturally high in cholesterol. Foods high in saturated fats include chocolate, tropical oils (that's why coconut oil–popped popcorn is bad news), and liquid oils other than olive oil or canola (a.k.a. rapeseed) oil. Now olive oil and canola oil do contain saturated fats, but they have a higher smoking temperature than other liquid oils, which helps reduce the fat.

Modern milk

We consume a lot of milk in North America. In the United States, each person consumes roughly 350 pounds of milk per year, which is equal to roughly 72 gallons of milk. That translates into one cow for every second person. However, the heating procedures, homogenization, sterilization, addition of other ingredients such as vitamin D, hormones, antibodies, and other chemicals in milk have led many people to wonder if milk is still nature's perfect food. When you consider that 75 percent of all dairy cows are artificially inseminated, milk somehow loses its wholesome aura.

The interesting thing about modern milk is that before we were able to store and preserve milk, the consumption of dairy products was limited to fermented dairy foods such as yogurt and kefir, which contain enzymes and bacteria that help us break down the dairy component.

Animal milk (from the goat, sheep, or donkey) was once reserved for mothers who couldn't breastfeed, but nature never intended humans to consume the huge quantities of animal milk that they do today.

Since it's probably not very practical to stop consuming all dairy products, here's the lowdown on milk products, so you can decide what to drop:

- Whole milk gets 48 percent of its calories from fat.
- 2 percent milk gets 37 percent of its calories from fat.
- 1 percent milk gets 26 percent of its calories from fat.
- Skim milk is completely fat-free.
- Cheese gets 50 percent of its calories from fat, unless it's skim milk cheese.
- Butter gets 95 percent of its calories from fat.
- Yogurt gets 15 percent of its calories from fat.

TRIMMING THE FAT

The best way to cut your dietary fat is to read labels. A product that boasts it has fewer calories can be low in sodium or low in sugar, but not necessarily low fat. Labels that scream "lower in fat" generally don't clarify what the product is being compared to. Anything would be lower than lard or butter. If you read a label that says "no cholesterol," it probably means that the product contains no animal fats, but could it contain saturated fats such as vegetable oil, which will raise your cholesterol levels anyway. Other label tricks include lowering the serving size. For instance, I actually fell for a label that screamed "only 89 calories" in big fat letters on potato crispy somethings. After I had consumed a good portion of the box, I realized it was 89 calories per "suggested serving" of six potato crisps (which, incidentally, weren't even made from real potatoes!).

Some of the most fattening products are sold as health foods: granola bars (200 calories, with roughly 50 percent derived from fat) and carob and yogurt candies. Even low-fat frozen yogurt can be high in fat, especially if you have it topped with fattening goodies.

"Good fat" isn't as hard to find as you think. Any of these are considered good fats: whole grains, beans, nuts, seeds, and the "good oils" mentioned earlier.

What you probably know . . . but may not

I hate to sound like your mother, but please remember that broiling, baking, steaming, poaching, roasting, or microwaving foods is healthier than frying or deep-frying. (I *know* you know this, but this is my job!)

Vegetables are good steamed, even boiled. Apparently, boiled vegetables are now thought to contain a thermoresistant substance that may have a protective effect against certain cancers. Roasting vegetables is fine, too. Here are some more fat-fighting tips:

- Whenever you refrigerate animal fat (as in soups, stews, or curry dishes), skim the fat from the top before re-heating and re-serving. A gravy skimmer will also help skim fats—the spout pours from the bottom, which enables the oils and fats to coagulate on top. A wilted lettuce leaf is also a good tool for skimming fat from the top of cans or broths.

- To cut some fat out of canned goods (soups, tuna, etc.), pour the contents through a coffee filter first. You can also refrigerate the can first—this will make all the fat rise to the top, which you can skim before serving.

- Substitute something else for butter: yogurt (great on potatoes), low-fat cottage cheese, or jams and jellies. You can also blend half butter with half olive or canola oil to create your own lower-calorie spread. Or, at dinner, just dip your bread in olive oil and garlic—Italian style. For sandwiches, any condiment without butter, margarine, or mayonnaise is fine—mustard, yogurt, etc.

- Powdered non-fat milk is in vogue again; it is high in calcium and low in fat. Substitute it for any recipe calling for milk or cream.

- Dig out fruit recipes for dessert. Things like sorbet (not to be confused with sherbet) with low-fat yogurt topping can be elegant. Sherbet is made with cream; sorbet is not.

- Season low-fat foods well. That way, you won't miss the flavor fat adds.

- Good carbohydrates are found in products with polysaccharide glucose (cereal, grains, veggies, beans); bad carbohydrates in monosaccharide or disaccharide sugars (fruit, honey, dairy foods, refined sugar, other sweeteners). Use this information to make better choices.

- Good protein comes from vegetable sources (whole grains and bean products); bad proteins come from animal sources. Again, use this information to make better choices.

Talk turkey

Many North Americans are substituting red meat for low-fat turkey meat. It's a good start. If you have to have beef, keep in mind that it varies in fat content. Prime beef carries the highest fat content; choice has less; select has the least. Lean beef is apparently an oxymoron, since beef isn't bred to be lean.

WHAT COLOR ARE YOUR VEGETABLES?

Nutritionist, fitness practitioner, and nurse Karen Faye explained to me the complex world of veggies. She categorized vegetables in her own sensible system for people like me who can never remember their vitamin ABCs. All green vegetables are for cellular repair (broccoli, green beans, spinach, lettuces, etc). All red, orange, yellow, and even purple vegetables contain antioxidants, which are thought to be cancer-fighting "GIs."

The theory of antioxidants, for those of us who need a refresher, goes like this: Cancer will thrive in oxygen-depleted cells or in an environment where carcinogens, radioactive particles, and other toxic wastes accumulate. We need oxygen to metabolize our food properly and to produce strong blood cells. In fact, without sufficient amounts of oxygen, we can't make efficient use of our calories. That's where antioxidants come in: they help distribute oxygen to the body, enabling it to use calories more efficiently. Antioxidants are found in fresh vegetables high in vitamins A, C, and E. So from now on, any vegetable with yellow, orange, red, or purple hues is a really good choice. Scientists also believe that foods high in soy, as well as broccoli, cabbage, and brussels sprouts promote the "good estrogen" (see Chapter 1), and inhibit the "bad estrogen," which may offer some protection.

A word about vitamin pills

Vitamins tend to work best when they're consumed with whole foods and other nutrients. The National Academy of Sciences reported that vitamin supplements can be toxic in high doses. So, it is better to focus on eating well than getting your vitamins from pills.

Greetings from Gilroy

Every year in California the Gilroy Garlic festival celebrates the wonders of garlic. In addition to fighting yeast infections, certain compounds found in garlic may help inhibit the growth of tumor cells. This is still just a theory, though. Garlic is also known to lower blood pressure.

Turning Japanese

Eating more sushi or other seaweed dishes is a good idea, too. Studies show that in Japan, where sea vegetables make up 1 percent of the diet, women are nine times less likely to develop postmenopausal breast cancer than their American friends, and three times less likely to develop premenopausal breast cancer than Americans. Studies also show that green tea, often served in Japanese restaurants and available in health food stores and even in brand name iced teas, can also help prevent cancer via a chemical it contains known as cathchin. Green tea also inhibits urokinase, an enzyme crucial for cancer growth.

LOCATION, LOCATION, LOCATION

Nutritionists also point out that a sensible diet has a lot to do with the ecology and environment surrounding you. In other words, the right diet is based on where you live. Traditional Inuit diets, for example, were based on animal products because of the low temperatures, which fat helped to combat. In hotter climates, such as in India and other tropical regions, lighter diets based on grains and vegetables, and even certain spices, were more conducive to good health.

Once we begin to eat food out of season and "off location," the food apparently loses some of the natural immunity it can provide when eaten freshly picked. Unfortunately, there's not much we can do about this, given that most of us live in urban areas. But it is important to be aware of this issue. Advances in refrigeration and transport have made it possible for us to eat as though we are in the tropics, and for people in the tropics to consume far more meat and dairy. Eastern nutritionists advise against foods that are not in "harmony" with the seasons. In cold weather, food that is cooked longer (soups and stews, for example) is considered better than salads and tropical fruits; while in summer, lighter fare is better than heavy meats and starches.

WHAT ABOUT ENVIRONMENTAL TOXINS?

As discussed in Chapter 1, there is currently a theory (which many medical experts believe is tenuous at best) that environmental toxins—particularly organic chemicals such as organochlorines—are associated with hormonal disruption in humans, contributing to diseases such as breast cancer, ovarian cancer, endometrial cancer, male reproductive cancers, endometriosis, and fibroids.

What can we do about this?

Right now, the only hope you and I have of eliminating these toxins (if, indeed they are as toxic as some say) is through consumer lobbying. Trend Number Eight in Faith Popcorn's 1991 *The Popcorn Report* is what she calls "The Vigilante Consumer." It's a trend corporate North America fears, and one that is fueling breast cancer activism all over the world.

THE GHOST OF LOBBYING PAST

Here are a few little inspirational ditties to get you thinking. Remember when Meryl Streep held a press conference to alert mothers like herself about how toxic apples treated with Alar (a type of pesticide) were? The issue turned into a cover story in *Newsweek,* which revealed that 6,000 American children could get cancer from ingesting produce with chemical residues such as those found on Alar-treated apples. The result? Alar was banned.

Everyman Phil Sokoloff spoke out against tropical oils in cereals and cookies because tropical oils are much higher in saturated fats. Companies like Keebler, General Mills, Borden, Pillsbury, Quaker Oats, Pepperidge Farm, and Kellogg removed tropical oils from their cereals and cookies. There are hundreds of examples just like that—including the movie theater popcorn "scandal," in which theatres were found to be popping their corn in coconut oil (which is much higher in fat and very unhealthy). This practice was halted thanks to consumers.

And we have the power to break businesses, too. Remember Perrier water? Just to refresh your memory, when Perrier was found to be neither natural (it was contaminated with benzene) nor naturally bubbly (seems as though the carbonation was factory-produced in New Jersey), Perrier lost its consumer confidence and was pulled out of the market for a long time.

Who can forget McDonald's response to consumer complaints about fluorocarbons in its Styrofoam packaging? It changed, too. How about that "dolphin safe" tuna (thanks to moms and kids who complained), plus the other consumer wins?

The bottom line is that since far more consumers of environmental toxins are concerned than the manufacturers of these toxins, it is up to people like you and me to make our concerns, *their* concerns. If you complain, they will change.

Food for thought

The best place to start the environmental "clean-up" is in your kitchen, with your weekly groceries. The store-bought fruits and vegetables probably contain residues from pesticides and other organochlorines; meat products contain hormones, as well as a number of "extras" you may not have bargained for that were fed to the animal when it was still alive. These include feed additives, antibiotics, and tranquilizers. Meanwhile, anything that is packaged will most likely contain dyes and flavors from a variety of chemical concoctions.

Airborne contaminants, waste, and spills affect the water and soil, which affects virtually everything we ingest. In addition, when one species becomes unable to reproduce, the food chain is interrupted, eventually affecting the food that reaches our kitchen tables. Cleaning up the food chain is part of creating a healthy, contaminant-free diet for ourselves. So make the following grocery list before your next shopping trip:

- You can find out what your meat produce has ingested and whether it was injected with anything by calling the USDA information line at 202-720-2791. (In Canada, call Agriculture and Agrafood Canada at 613-952-8000).
- You can find out what waters your fish swam in by calling the numbers listed above.
- You can find "safe food" that is organically grown through a number of natural produce supermarkets (such as Bread and Circus, for example).

- You can find out what your grown produce was sprayed with by calling the numbers listed above.
- You can find out more about your supermarket's buying habits when it comes to produce by contacting your supermarket's head office.

Since the origin of the word *consumer* comes from the word *consume* (to eat), becoming vigilant about our groceries is the only way we can help change the produce and food stuff industry. Customers are incredibly powerful to any company. In the 1980s, it was the "vigilante consumer" who helped to make manufacturers more green-friendly and value-conscious. In many instances, the sheer volume of customer complaints and letters has completely changed not only an individual company's habits and policies, but that of the entire industry. If enough customers ban products and protest manufacturing or agricultural practices, the companies will change. Bring new meaning to the adage, "the customer is always right."

Read any good labels, lately?

Worried about the plastic that lines certain canned goods? Demand labeling that identifies the organic chemicals used to make that plastic. Worried about the plastics used in various cosmetics, detergents, spermicides? Write letters to manufacturers; call 1-800 numbers; start a newsgroup on the Internet; lobby; protest; ban products to help change standards. Don't be afraid to write letters to the editors of daily newspapers or to call for press conferences on various labeling, packaging, or ingredient issues that concern you. What exactly is plastic wrap made out of, anyway? You have a right to know. What was this spinach sprayed with? You have a right to a label that reads: "This produce sprayed with endosulfan." To date, the chemical ingredients in plastic products are kept from the consumer because they are considered "trade secrets." This is unacceptable. As consumers, we must use our collective voice to help get labeling details on the containers that house our produce, as well as the breeders that bred our produce. Perhaps Faith Popcorn put it best when she predicted that by 2010:

Labels will become more important than ever before. We'll want to know (like Big Brother) a biography of the product and the ethics of the maker. We'll want to know the company's stand on the environment, how it regards animal testing, human rights, and other issues—rather than just a list of ingredients or a glimpse of an image. Listed prominently on the label, 800 numbers connecting the consumer to the corporation will be a way of life. (*The Popcorn Report* by Faith Popcorn, Doubleday, 1991, page 77.)

WHAT YOUR GOVERNMENT IS DOING

In 1958, the United States government passed an amendment to the federal Food, Drug and Cosmetic Act. Called the Delaney Clause, the amendment was designed to protect the public from residues of carcinogenic pesticides in processed foods and called for an absolute ban on these chemicals. But in 1965, the National Academy of Sciences (NAS) concluded that an absolute ban was not scientifically realistic, and the Delaney Clause was abandoned. Ever since, the Food and Drug Administration and the Department of Agriculture have set "allowable" levels of chemicals in our food.

In the late 1980s, the Environmental Protection Agency (EPA) in the United States established "negligible risk tolerances" for all carcinogenic pesticides on all foods. But this particular risk assessment doesn't consider the *cumulative* effects of possible cancer-causing pesticides in our diet, drinking water, and air. In other words, it does not assess how many "hits" our cells can take of these pesticides before turning cancerous.

By 1992, the EPA was ordered to remove food with pesticide residue from supermarket shelves. This helped to get the National Cancer Institute to at least begin to study the effects of environmental contaminants

To date, the International Joint Commission, which is an advisory body on environmental issues, has recommended to the United States and Canadian governments that organochlorines be phased out as a class, not simply on a chemical-by-chemical basis.

In the meantime, put pressure on your local members of government as well as your medical community to:

- caution people about the possible dangers of estrogenic toxins found in pesticides, foods, gasoline, car emissions, synthetic estrogens and even some anti-depressant drugs
- encourage all women and caution pregnant women to breastfeed their children and avoid home use of pesticides
- urge the World Health Organization to stop recommending the use of DDT
- urge regulatory bodies to test how chemicals and drugs impact our reproductive systems before they grant approval
- refrain from using diagnostic x-rays in children, especially girls, unless absolutely necessary
- encourage low-fat eating and regular physical activity at young ages in all public and private schools

MEDICAL PREVENTION STRATEGIES

Therapies and intervention from the medical community are another aspect of breast cancer prevention that is worth examining. As of this writing, experts predict that we are still about ten years away from safe and effective breast cancer prevention therapies, however.

GENETIC TESTING

As discussed in Chapter 1, you can be tested for the breast cancer gene BRCA1 (BRCA2 will be available by 1997). But while BRCA1 and BRCA2 account for roughly 90 percent of all inherited breast cancer (accounting for 5 to 10 percent of all breast cancers), their role in non-inherited breast cancer is not known.

If you have inherited a *mutated* form of either gene, you have an 80 to 90 percent risk of getting breast cancer by age 85, compared to the 12 percent risk the general population faces. Testing positive for the gene is meaningless unless you have a strong family history of breast cancer, however.

There is much discussion over genetic testing and insurance coverage. Would testing positive affect your coverage the way testing positive for HIV often does? While several states don't allow genetic test results to have any weight when it comes to coverage and premiums, this rule is not applicable when health insurance comes through an employer.

That's not to say that research into genes doesn't hold promise. If scientists can find a way to replace a defective BRCA1 or BRCA2 gene with a normal one, than we might have a real way of preventing breast cancer (this technology is still ten years away, however). See Chapter 1 for more information on genetic testing.

TAMOXIFEN: THE TRIAL OF THE CENTURY

Tamoxifen—the very same drug used in hormone breast cancer therapy (see Chapter 4)—is being studied as a possible prevention drug for breast cancer in women considered at high risk for the disease (women who come from families with a high incidence of bilateral breast cancer in first-degree relatives are currently considered at high risk). The use of tamoxifen as prevention therapy is extremely controversial because tamoxifen is an anti-estrogen drug, which means that it would have side effects when given to healthy women without any sign of breast cancer, and these side effects need to be weighed against the perceived benefits of this drug. Critics of the tamoxifen prevention trial (and there are many) argue that the trial is motivated by profit. If the trial shows that tamoxifen can help prevent breast cancer, then, in theory, one half of the population becomes the target market.

In 1992, $70 million was allocated to the tamoxifen breast cancer prevention study. The study at that point involved giving tamoxifen to 8,000 women at random, while another 8,000 would be put on a placebo. The women on tamoxifen were administered the same dosage as women in treatment who were fighting breast cancer. Critics of the trial argued that these women were not informed of the side effects tamoxifen has below the waist: menopausal symptoms and endometrial and liver cancer (one to three out of a thousand women will develop endometrial cancer, which is a very small risk). The trial's recruitment criteria was also criticized; 98.2 percent of all women recruited were white, coloring any meaningful data for women of other ethnic origins.

So far, more than 40,000 women worldwide have signed up for various tamoxifen trials—all designed to study the long-term impact of giving a synthetic anti-estrogen drug to otherwise healthy women at high risk for breast cancer.

The side effects issue

Since tamoxifen can cause liver cancer and endometrial cancer in roughly one to three in a thousand, it has polarized the medical community into tamoxifen supporters and tamoxifen opponents. The supporters see prevention of breast cancer as a victory that outweighs the side effects of tamoxifen such as blood clots (also a risk for women on the pill), depression, and the small risks of endometrial cancer and liver cancer. The opponents of tamoxifen feel that it is unethical to administer a powerful anti-estrogen drug to healthy women—even if they are supposedly at high risk for breast cancer. Again, as explained in Chapter 1, only 30 percent of all breast cancers develop in women with known risk factors, 5 percent of these in women with a family history of breast cancer.

Are you a candidate?

Technically, the FDA hasn't approved tamoxifen as a preventive drug for breast cancer. Despite this, many doctors will prescribe it to patients they consider high risk for breast cancer as part of the tamoxifen trial. High risk, in this case, means you have a mother or sister who had or has bilateral breast cancer prior to menopause. If you have an aunt who developed breast cancer after sixty-five, however, you are not considered at high risk; this is simply taken as family history.

How does it work?

No one really knows exactly why tamoxifen works on breast cancer but the current theory is that by interfering with estrogen, which is what makes most breast cancer cells "go," tamoxifen inhibits the cancer cells from growing further—or, in the case of a preventive measure, from growing at all. Tamoxifen has therefore been used as a treatment for breast cancer both advanced and early-stage for the past twenty years.

But because it is a powerful anti-estrogen, tamoxifen's effect on still-healthy women is also powerful. In addition, tamoxifen is only effective in estrogen-dependent breast cancer, which only accounts for about one-third of all breast tumors. Some tamoxifen critics argue that the drug may stimulate non-estrogen tumors to grow in the breast, but there is no conclusive proof of this. Another point of contention is the age of the tamoxifen recipient. While the drug has been proven effective in treating postmenopausal women, it hasn't been proven effective in premenopausal women. But the only women enrolled in the tamoxifen trials are premenopausal.

What are the side effects?

Since tamoxifen is an anti-estrogen, it usually leads to menopausal side effects that are associated with estrogen "withdrawal." These include irregular periods, hot flashes, and vaginal dryness. Other side effects include weight gain, mild to severe depression, and "cold" flashes. There is also a risk of blood clots (also a risk with hormonal contraceptives), endometrial cancer, and liver cancer (again, this is considered a very small risk).

In Italy, tamoxifen is reserved only for women who have had hysterectomies because of the risk of endometrial cancer. Apparently, studies show that tamoxifen-related endometrial cancer can be more severe than other forms of endometrial cancer.

Some studies show a link on rare occasions to severe vision problems and blindness. In fact, clomiphene citrate, a fertility drug, is also known for causing severe vision problems.

If you're thinking about tamoxifen, use the pill guidelines to help you decide. For example, if you're at risk for blood clots, if you smoke, or may be pregnant, don't go anywhere *near* this drug. In addition, if you're on oral contraceptives or other hormonal contraceptives such as Norplant or Depo-Provera, you must not take tamoxifen unless you stop these medications first. And if you're wearing an IUD (intrauterine device), it must come out before you start tamoxifen. Tamoxifen can cause your uterine lining to thicken, which is why there's a risk of endometrial cancer—wearing an IUD could greatly complicate matters.

If you're thinking of enrolling in a tamoxifen study or are offered the drug by your doctor, be sure to have a full physical exam before you make your decision. This includes checking your blood levels and having a pelvic exam, a breast exam, and possibly a mammogram—and an electrocardiogram (ECG) if you're over fifty-five.

OTHER PREVENTION DRUGS

Unlikely breast cancer prevention drugs that have recently surfaced are aspirin (ASA) and non-steroidal, anti-inflammatory drugs (NSAIDs) such as ibuprofen. It's been shown that women who regularly use ASA or NSAIDs may reduce the risk of breast cancer. And, by increasing usage of ASA and NSAIDs, women newly diagnosed with breast cancer may see smaller tumors and less lymph node involvement. NSAIDs work by inhibiting prostaglandins, the hormone that makes things "flare up" in our bodies. That's why NSAIDs are used so often to help relieve arthritis or menstrual cramps. Well, it's been found that prostaglandins play a role in cancer cell growth, too, which is why NSAIDs appear to work. In one analysis of breast cancer patients, at least 60 percent of those who took ten or more NSAID or aspirin pills per month had tumors smaller than two centimeters and lymph node involvement. Many oncologists feel that NSAIDs and aspirin should begin to be used right now as ways to help prevent breast cancer. As for dosage, check with your doctor; this is very new and guidelines haven't come out yet.

Currently, hormones are being looked at as a way to kill to two birds with one stone: lowering the risk of breast cancer while providing contraception. Injecting women with a pituitary hormone currently used for fertility treatment (gonadotropin releasing hormone or GnRH), into which research is ongoing, is being seen by some as an advancement in preventive therapy. GnRH would be injected monthly, followed by estrogen and progesterone. Of course, this kind of preventive treatment will serve to polarize the prevention camps even more.

PREVENTIVE MASTECTOMY

Discussed briefly in previous chapters, preventive or prophylactic mastectomy is sometimes recommended by doctors, although this is pretty rare. Surgeons I've interviewed tell me that this procedure is done when the patient wants it, rather than the doctor. While this kind of mastectomy does lower your risk, it can't guarantee that you'll never get breast cancer because some breast tissue remains. In any event, these are the only scenarios where this procedure should ever be considered:

- Risk of bilateral, premenopausal familial breast cancer. For example, if your mother and sister both developed bilateral invasive breast cancer at, say, age thirty-five, you would be considered very likely to develop breast cancer around this age, too. Studies show that younger women in their twenties or early thirties have the most to gain by prophylactic mastectomy in these circumstances, but women sixty or older haven't much to gain.
- Diagnosis of lobular carcinoma in situ (a marker for breast cancer risk, discussed in Chapter 3). Lobular carcinoma in situ (LCIS) is considered a sign of higher cancer risk in either breast. Depending on your age and your medical and family history, preventive mastectomy may be an option.
- Breast cancer has been diagnosed in one breast. Depending on the staging and invasiveness of the cancer, a preventive mastectomy for the other breast may be an option.

The decision to have a preventive mastectomy is highly individual. Since the advent of far more sensitive mammograms (which will presumably get more sensitive as time goes on), many experts are abandoning preventive mastectomy as a prevention strategy. So if preventive mastectomy is being recommended, you should definitely seek out a second opinion from a breast surgeon (not just a general surgeon). See Chapter 3 for more information.

BREAST CANCER EDUCATION

"Early detection is your best protection" is how most women think of breast cancer education. That's still true today, but there is much more education that needs to get out to your daughters and granddaughters about risk (Chapter 1), screening and investigation (Chapter 2), diagnosis and treatment decisions (Chapters 3 and 4), and ways to be proactive about our health (see the beginning of this chapter), which includes modifying our diets. Education is the key to the future of this disease, since it is increasing, not decreasing.

Suppose your daughters were required to complete a breast education unit in their high schools as part of their health class. They are currently required to take sex education (although the curriculum is much in debate these days), which teaches them about safe sex and HIV prevention. The curriculum of a breast education unit would include breast self-exam and would also discuss the role of genetics, diet, and the environment in breast cancer risk. Perhaps your daughter might make certain decisions about her diet while she is young, perhaps she might even become an early "pro" at doing breast self-exams, and she may become a more thoughtful consumer when it comes to risks associated with environmental factors. It's also important that educators help daughters of breast cancer patients get the necessary counseling to deal with their own risk profile. Studies not only show that these young women grossly overestimate their risk of breast cancer, but during their mothers' illnesses, they can become very distressed and martyr-like, dropping out of school, for example, to care for their mothers. These women are also far more likely to suffer from lifelong depressive or anxiety disorders.

Or what if breast cancer education was made available to *you* in a variety of forums: Lunch & Learn programs at various companies; malls; public service announcements with a 1-800 number made available; print ads and billboards. Would it be helpful? Do you think this is worth considering for other women?

Indeed, future trends in health care point to more corporations shouldering more responsibility for prevention initiatives. Corporations which *depend* on women's dollars or women's *labor*, such as retailers, airlines, or pharmaceutical companies who make women's health products, are ideal sponsors for spreading breast cancer education among the masses. People like you and me who work for such corporations are in a good position to suggest education programs like these.

ACTIVISM AND EDUCATION

In case you've forgotten, it took a lot of activism by AIDS organizations for AIDS to be taken seriously by legislators and the research community. Nobody wanted to be associated with a disease that infected (at first) gay men. And the public health disaster that largely resulted from procrastination and disinterest on the part of the health industry is a reality that millions of people worldwide might have avoided if the right steps were taken at the right time.

Many women see breast cancer as an ignored epidemic that is only getting worse, since even the causes of breast cancer remain uncertain. Women have learned a valuable lesson from AIDS activists and are now lobbying and organizing themselves from the grassroots up, instead of the top down.

Reporter Linda Ellerbee put it well when she described the difference between AIDS and breast cancer. While AIDS is always fatal, she pointed out, many women survive breast cancer. This fact has seemed to make AIDS more of a priority for funding and research (quite the opposite of what it used to be), while breast cancer seems to have been left behind in many respects.

But what's happened is that breast cancer is no longer a disease that our mothers and grandmothers had. It's killing children of the 1950s and 1960s: you and me. As a result, we're seeing these generations tackle breast cancer in the same way they tackled civil rights and the women's movement: activism.

One of the best examples of breast cancer activism is 1 in 9, started in Long Island by a group of women who were, for lack of a better phrase, "pissed off" that breast cancer rates were higher in their community than in other parts of New York.

One in 9 was started in 1987 when teacher and grandmother Francine Kritchek and the late Marie Quinn, a friend of Francine's who also had breast cancer, sent out a letter about the disease to everyone in their school. But when a state study of Long Island's breast cancer rates found a relationship between high breast cancer incidence and high levels of household income, but did not even look into environmental factors, Kritchek and Quinn got mad. They contacted two other women, put an ad in the paper, and sent a mailing to hundreds of people announcing a meeting. Before long, 1 in 9 was established. Fifty-seven angry women showed up at the first meeting, and 300 women protested in front of a Long Island court.

Now there are well over one hundred eighty advocacy groups, including 1 in 9, that are united under the National Breast Cancer Coalition, a volunteer-driven organization that was founded in 1991. These activists are not only demanding more money for breast cancer research but want to help guide *where* the money goes. That will help to fund some truly significant research into this disease.

The National Breast Cancer Coalition was able to increase research funding into breast cancer by $43 million in 1991—an increase of almost 50 percent over 1990. By 1992, the coalition was able to get $300 million more for research, helped in part by data from a seminar it funded. When the National Breast Cancer Coalition delivered 600,000 signatures to Washington on Breast Cancer Awareness Day in 1992, they were able to win some friends. Then Iowa Senator Tom Harkin introduced the coalition to the U.S. Department of Defense; in the end, the U.S. Army's $25 million in funds for screening women in uniform was increased to $210 million and used for breast cancer research.

What is this activism doing for you?

Is all this activist-driven research money going to a good cause? Well, it depends on whom you talk to. Members of the National Breast Cancer Coalition want their money to research a cure for breast cancer once and for all. But there are hundreds of areas that surround finding a cure, from understanding how breast cancer cells work and behave so we can find drugs to kill those cancer cells, to developing stronger forms of chemotherapy and hormone therapy with fewer side effects.

Brigham and Women's Hospital in Boston reported in early 1995 that it was on the verge of discovering peptides that could one day help in the development of a vaccine against breast cancer and ovarian cancer; the peptide somehow induced immunity to these cancers. In the fall of 1996, encouraging studies surfaced about making chemotherapy more effective by testing the drugs that work on your cancer cells in a lab *before* administering your chemotherapy.

Many scientists feel that the cure for breast cancer lies in reversing the earliest genetic mutations of the disease—an area into which there is considerable research. Some feel that more research should go into understanding more about the environmental causes of breast cancer (food, air, lifestyle, culture, and so on).

Activist-raised money may also help to fund free mammograms and manual breast exams in the United States for women who currently can't afford medical care, while women in countries with universal health care will benefit from breast health awareness education programs.

EXTRAS AND GOODIES

In the final pages of this chapter, you'll find some useful tables from my "odds and ends" file that I wanted to share with you. If you've managed to sort through all the information in this chapter (not to mention the rest of the book)—you deserve a reward! Of particular interest is table 10.5, which reminds us that with the bitter, there is also the sweet.

• • • • • • •

Since I know so many of you will be reading this part of the book first, I'll tell you what's inside these pages. This is a book that deals with breast cancer risk (Chapter 1), detection and screening (Chapter 2), diagnosis and treatment (Chapters 3 through 9), and prevention (this chapter). Whether you're worried about your risk of developing breast cancer down the road or have just felt a lump in the shower and don't know what it is yet or have been actually diagnosed with breast cancer, you'll find a lot of the information you need now, and probably more than you want to know.

If you're in the middle of breast treatment, go directly to Chapter 3. From there on, you'll find the rest of the book is designed for you and your family.

There are some chapters that deal with special concerns, as well. Chapter 5 discusses breast reconstruction and alternatives; Chapter 6 discusses unique concerns of lovers and spouses of women with breast cancer; Chapter 7 discusses complementary medicine; while Chapter 9 discusses palliative care.

You'll find a detailed resource list I've called "breastcancer.com," with comprehensive directions for using the Internet to find even more resources and information.

But most important, I want to hear from you. What information is missing that you need? How can I make this a more useful book for you in future editions? How has this book helped you? Please write to me care of the publisher. If you're a woman age eighteen or over, I promise you haven't been left out of this sourcebook. Share it with your mothers, grandmothers, daughters, and grand-daughters. And, by all means, take this book with you to your doctors' appointments. I wish you luck. I wish you good health. And I wish you peace of mind.

Table 10.1
AMERICAN MEDICAL ASSOCIATION GUIDELINES

Though not directed specifically at cancer, the American Medical Association issued dietary guidelines to reduce the overall risk of degenerative disease:

1. Eat meat no more than once a day and choose fish or poultry over red meat.
2. Bake or broil food rather than frying it and use polyunsaturated oils rather than butter, lard, or margarine.
3. Cut down on salt, MSG, and other flavorings high in sodium.
4. Eat more fiber, including whole-grain cereals, leafy green vegetables, and fruit.
5. Eat no more than four eggs a week.
6. For dessert or a snack, eat fruit rather than baked goods.

In a review of special diets, the nation's medical association advised:

In the macrobiotic diet foods fall into two main groups, known as yin and yang (based on an Eastern principle of opposites), depending on where they have been grown, their texture, color, and composition. The general principle behind this diet is that foods biologically furthest away from us are better for us. Cereals, therefore, form the basis of the diet and fish is preferred over meat. Although fresh foods free of additives are preferred, no food is actually prohibited, in the belief that a craving for any food may reflect a genuine bodily need. In general, the macrobiotic diet is a healthful way of eating. However, extreme adherents of macrobiotics restrict fluid intake, and this could be harmful to health.

Source: Kushi, Michio. The Cancer Prevention Guide. New York: St. Martins Press, 1993: 447.

Table 10.2
COMPARISON OF CHINESE AND AMERICAN DIETS

Dietary intakes	China	U.S.
Total Dietary fiber (g/day)	33.3	11.1
Starch (g/day)	371	120
Plant protein (% of total)	89	30
Fat (% of calories)	14.5	38.8
Calcium (mg/day)	544	1143
Retinol (vit. A equiv/day)	27.8	990
Total carotenoids (retinol equiv/day)	836	429
Vitamin C (mg/day)	140	73
Blood plasma constituents		
Cholesterol (mg/dl)	127	212
Triglycerides (mg/dl)	97	120
Total protein (g/dl)	4.8–6.2	6.4–8.3

Source: Kushi, Michio. The Cancer Prevention Guide. *New York: St. Martins Press, 1993: 450.*

Table 10.3
CANCER-INHIBITING SUBSTANCES IN BASIC MACROBIOTIC FOODS

Foods	Cancer-inhibiting factors
Whole grains	Fiber, protease inhibitors, vitamin E
Beans	Fiber, protease inhibitors, vitamin E
Miso, tofu, tempeh, and other soy foods	Isoflavones, protease inhibitors, phytosterols, saponins, phytoestrogens
Green leafy vegetables	Beta-carotene, and other carotenoid pigments, chlorophyll, fiber, vitamins A, C, and E
Orange-yellow vegetables	Beta-carotene and other carotenoid pigments, fiber, vitamins A and C
Cruciferous vegetables	Indoles, dithiolthiones, glucosinolates, carotenoids, chlorophyll, fiber, vitamins A, C, and E
Sea vegetables	Fiber, chlorophyll, fucoidan, vitamin C

Source: Kushi, Michio. The Cancer Prevention Guide. *New York: St. Martins Press, 1993: 51.*

Table 10.4

AMERICAN CANCER SOCIETY GUIDELINES ON DIET, NUTRITION, AND CANCER

In 1984, the American Cancer Society issued guidelines for the first time on diet and cancer, calling for increased consumption of high-fiber foods such as whole grains and fresh vegetables and fruits. In 1991 the society updated its recommendations noting:

Evidence from numerous experimental and human population studies conducted during past years suggests that a large proportion of human cancers may be associated with what we eat an drink and certain other lifestyle factors. It is estimated that about one-third of the annual 500,000 deaths from cancer in the United States, including the most common sites such as breast, colon, and prostate, may be attributed to undesirable dietary practice. . . .

Recommendations:

1. Maintain a desirable body weight.
2. Eat a varied diet.
3. Include a variety of both vegetables and fruits in the daily diet.
4. Eat more high-fiber foods, such as whole-grain cereals, legumes, vegetables, and fruits.
5. Cut down on total fat intake.
6. Limit consumption of alcoholic beverage, if you drink at all.
7. Limit consumption of salt-cured, smoked, and nitrite-preserved foods.

The guidelines noted:

- The consumption of vegetables and fruits is associated with a decreased risk of lung, prostate, bladder, esophagus, and stomach cancers.
- High fiber-containing vegetables, fruits, and cereals can be recommended as wholesome low-calorie substitutes for high-calorie fatty foods.
- For most healthy adults, a decrease in fat calories to 25 to 30 percent or less of total calories intake can be achieved by changes in eating habits to reduce the consumption of fats, oils, and foods rich in fats, such as fatty meats, whole-fat diary products, gravies, sauces, salad dressings, and high-fat desserts.

Source: Kushi, Michio. The Cancer Prevention Guide. New York: St. Martins Press, 1993: 446.

Table 10.5
SWEET SOMETHINGS

"Best Bites" get no more than: one gram of saturated fat, 20 percent of their calories from fat, and 60 percent of their calories from fat and sugar combined. They also contain at least 10 percent of the Daily Value (DV) for naturally occurring calcium, fiber, or vitamins A or C. "Honorable Mentions" met the fat, saturated fat, and sugar limits only.

Following each product's name (in parentheses) are the number of brownies, muffins, etc., or the portion of a cake, pie, or mix that makes one serving. Products in bold are full-fat versions for comparison. Within each category, products are ranked from lowest percent of calories from fat to highest, before rounding.

Item	Calories	Calories from fat (%)	Total fat (g)	Calories from sugar (%)
Cakes (1½ to 3½ oz per serving)				
♦ Entenmann's Fat Free Banana or Blueberry Crunch[2] (⅛)	140	0	0	54
♦ Betty Crocker Fat Free Sweet Rewards Mix[1] (⅛)	170	0	0	55
♦ Entenmann's Fat Free Loaf[1] (⅛)	135	0	0	57
Entenmann's Fat Free Chocolate Crunch (⅛)	130	0	0	62
Entenmann's Fat Free Carrot (⅛)	170	0	0	64
Duncan Hines Angel Food Mix[1] (1/12)	130	0	0	68
Entenmann's Fat Free Fudge Iced Chocolate (⅙)	210	0	0	72
♦ Weight Watchers Chocolate Raspberry Royale (1)	190	14	3	46
♦ Healthy Oven Low-Fat Quick-Cake Mix[1] (1/9)	115	16	2	31
Betty Crocker Light SuperMoist Mix[1#] (1/10)	225	17	4	44
♦ Sara Lee Free & Light Pound Cake (¼)	200	18	4	42
Entenmann's 50% Less Fat Fudge Iced Golden[#] (⅙)	270	20	6	56
Entenmann's 50% Less Fat All Butter Loaf[#] (⅛)	140	23	4	40
Entenmann's 50% Less Fat All Butter Marble Loaf[#] (⅛)	150	24	4	37
Betty Crocker SuperMoist no-cholesterol recipe[1#] (1/12)	215	29	7	38
Entenmann's Chocolate Fudge[#] (⅙)	**310**	**41**	**14**	**45**
Sara Lee All Butter Pound Cake[#] (⅙)	**320**	**45**	**16**	**26**
Doughnuts, Danish, Coffee Cake, and Buns (about 2 oz. per serving)				
♦ Entenmann's Fat Free Cinnamon Apple Coffee Cake (1/9)	130	0	0	49

continued on next page

Table 10.5 *continued*

Item	Calories	Calories from fat (%)	Total fat (g)	Calories from sugar (%)
◆ Entenmann's Fat Free Buns[1] (1)	150	0	0	51
◆ Entenmann's Fat Free Twist[1]	145	0	0	55
◆ Entenmann's Fat Free Black Forest or Raspberry Cheese Pastry[2] (1/9)	135	0	0	55
◆ Entenmann's Fat Free Apple Spice Crumb Cakes (1)	190	17	4	51
Entenmann's 50% Less Fat Cheese Coffee Cake# (1/8)	140	23	4	40
Weight Watchers Glazed Cinnamon Rolls# (1)	200	23	5	20
Entenmann's 50% Less Fat All Butter French Crumb Cake# (1/8)	170	24	5	40
Entenmann's 50% Less Fat Donuts, Glazed# (1)	220	25	6	51
Pillsbury Reduced Fat Cinnamon Rolls (1)	140	26	4	26
Entenmann's 50% Less Fat Raspberry Danish Twist# (1/8)	170	26	5	38
Entenmann's 50% Less Fat Crumb Delight (1/9)	210	26	6	38
Entenmann's 50% Less Fat Donuts, Devil's Food Crumb# (1)	240	26	7	40
Weight Watchers Sweet Celebrations Chocolate Eclair# (1)	150	30	5	37
Entenmann's 40% Less Fat Cheese Filled Crumb Coffee Cake# (1/8)	180	30	6	33
Entenmann's 50% Less Fat Donuts, Powdered Sugar# (1)	180	30	6	36
Dunkin' Donuts Chocolate Frosted Donut# (1)	210	34	8	23
Entenmann's 50% Less Fat Donuts, Fantastic Fudge# (1)	210	39	9	34
Entenmann's Cinnamon Buns# (1)	**220**	**41**	**10**	**33**
Sara Lee Pecan Coffee Cake# (1/6)	**220**	**49**	**12**	**18**
Entenmann's Danish Ring# (1/5)	**220**	**53**	**13**	**16**
Entenmann's Cinnamon Sugar Donuts (1)	**310**	**55**	**19**	**22**
Dunkin' Donuts Old Fashioned Donut# (1)	**280**	**61**	**19**	**10**
Entenmann's Rich Frosted Donuts, Variety Pack size# (1)	**400**	**61**	**27**	**21**

◆ = Honorable Mention   [1] = Average for the entire line   [2] = Average for the items listed   # = Contains at least 2 g of saturated fat (after rounding). Information obtained from manufacturers. Some products are regional, and products and numbers may vary in Canada. The use of information from this article for commercial purposes is strictly prohibited without written permission from CSPI.

Source: Adapted from Nutrition Action Newsletter, January/February 1996.

GLOSSARY

abortion: the medical term for miscarriage, used particularly in medical papers

absolute risk: refers to the cancer rate counted in numbers of cases occurring within a group of people

adjuvant therapy: additional therapy following surgery even though it's not immediately indicated, with the aim of preventing recurrence; sometimes called "insurance" by cancer specialists, although it is *not* a guarantee against future recurrence (neo-adjuvant therapy refers to adjuvant therapy prior to surgery)

analgesic: painkiller

animal studies: studies using animals, *not* humans, and *not* necessarily primates; a key when reading about studies and risk in the media

anorexia: loss of appetite; a common symptom associated with many chemotherapy drugs or advanced cancer

antioxidants: found in fresh vegetables high in vitamins A, C, and E; they help distribute oxygen to the body; cancer will thrive in oxygen-depleted cells, and thus antioxidants are thought to help protect against cancer

association: when you see a sentence like "women with breast cancer were found to eat more fat than women without breast cancer," this is association, *not* causation

attributable risk: refers to a component of your risk attributable to some factors you can change, such as diet or smoking, and some factors you cannot change, such as family history

autologous blood transfusion: when you bank your own blood prior to surgery so that your own blood can be used if you require a transfusion

axillary dissection: removal of lymph nodes from the armpit area; *axilla* means armpit

benign: harmless or non-cancerous, as in benign tumor

bilateral: means both sides, as in bilateral breast cancer, bilateral mastectomy, or bilateral reconstruction

BRCA 1: the most well-known breast cancer gene that has been isolated; responsible for 4 percent of all breast cancer cases; women who have this gene are more susceptible to breast cancer than those who don't

brachytherapy (internal radiation): planting a piece of radioactive material directly inside a tumor

breast screening: screening healthy women for breast cancer

BSE (Breast Self-Exam): a procedure in which women eighteen and over inspect their breasts monthly by looking at them carefully and feeling them for unusual changes

CA 15-3: a blood test that detects breast cancer cell sheddings; currently being used to detect recurrence of a breast cancer

carcinogen: a cancer-causing agent or substance

carcinoma: a clump of cancerous cells

causation: when you see a sentence like "smoking causes lung cancer," this is causation

chemotherapy: treating a medical condition with drugs; cancer patients are treated with anti-cancer drugs, which involve a range of side effects (see table 4.1)

closely related cancers: breast, ovarian, endometrial, and uterine cancers are all hormone-related and thus considered "closely related"

complementary therapy: non-Western medicine practices, such as acupuncture, which may accompany Western therapies

connective tissue disease: an umbrella term used to describe a variety of aches and pains that some experts link to silicone implant rupture or leakage; studies to date do not show a link, however; sometimes called autoimmune disease because the symptoms mimic rheumatoid arthritis and/or lupus—which are both autoimmune diseases

contraindicated: when a drug or therapy is *not recommended* in conjunction with the presence of a particular medical history or condition or other drug therapy

cumulative risk: risk that's simply "added up"; a risk per unit of time added up over X units of time, such as a lifetime or a given time frame that a study ran

cyclical breast pain: premenstrual breast tenderness; the breast pain thus disappears after your period; non-cyclical breast pain is persistent breast pain that isn't connected to your menstrual cycle

cyst: a fluid-filled lump that is usually harmless, which can be collapsed through a needle biopsy

DDT: abbreviation for dichlorodiphenyltrichloroethane; a pesticide widely used by most industrialized countries and banned in North America in the 1970s; breaks down into the byproduct DDE.

DES: abbreviation for diethylstilbestrol; a drug administered to pregnant women from the 1940s to the 1970s with the aim of preventing miscarriage

diagnostic X rays: these emit very low doses of radiation and do *not* count as high-dose radiation

dietary fat: refers to fat you eat and can therefore control

differentiated: refers to the sophistication of the cancer cell: a well-differentiated cancer cell resembles the cells of its origin, while a poorly differentiated or undifferentiated cancer cell is more primitive and "wild" looking

ductal carcinoma (DCIS): when breast cancer originates in the breast ducts; can be in situ or invasive

early menarche: when a woman has her first period before age twelve (in North America)

electromagnetic fields: areas near power lines or high electricity; electric blankets are also sources of electromagnetic fields

endometrium: uterine lining; endometrial cancer refers to cancer of the uterine lining

environmental estrogens: manmade chemicals that mimic the female hormone estrogen when they break down in the environment; sometimes referred to as estrogen mimics or gender-bending chemicals

estrogen: female hormone secreted by the ovaries

estrogenic: a substance that mimics estrogen or has estrogen properties

false negative: when a test comes back negative but is really positive

false positive: when a test comes back positive but is really negative

family history: the medical history of family members

fibroadenoma: a very common, solid benign lump that feels like a marble inside your breast and is often very close to the nipple

fibrocystic breast condition: an umbrella term that refers to separate and distinct breast conditions, ranging from premenstrual tenderness to cysts; formerly called fibrocystic breast disease, which is now an outdated label

first-degree relatives: immediate family members—parents, siblings, and children; grandmothers, aunts, and paternal relatives are not first-degree relatives

fluid accumulation: a condition that often occurs when cancer spreads to the lungs and blocks the lymph nodes that drain the area, resulting in shortness of breath and sharp chest pain

grading: refers to how well or poorly differentiated a cancer cell is

HDL ("good" cholesterol): the initials for high-density lipids

high-dose radiation: this includes high-dose X rays such as fluoroscopy

high-risk family: if you come from a family in which more than one first-degree relative has had breast cancer, you come from a high-risk family

HRT: the initials for hormone replacement therapy, which refers to the progesterone and estrogen given to women after menopause to prevent symptoms of estrogen loss; women with no uterus are given only estrogen

hormone therapy: usually involves therapy with an estrogen-blocking drug; used in breast cancer patients whose cancer cells are estrogen-receptor positive

hyperprolactinemia: oversecretion of the hormone prolactin, which in turn can inhibit estrogen production

in situ: a cancer that's in one place; non-invasive by definition

invasive: a cancer that can spread to local tissue, surrounding tissue, lymph nodes, or other organs

known risk factors: accounting for less than 30 percent of all breast cancers

lactation: when the breast is producing milk

lactational mastitis: a bacterial infection of a milk-producing breast, causing soreness, redness, and flu-like symptoms; you would have to be breastfeeding to get this

late menarche: when a woman has her first period after age seventeen (in North America)

LDL ("bad" cholesterol): the initials for low-density lipids

lobular carcinoma: when breast cancer originates in the lobes

lobular carcinoma in situ (LCIS): this is not considered a cancer, but simply a marker that a woman is at increased risk of developing invasive breast cancer—in the ducts or in the lobes—at some future date

local recurrence: a recurrence of the first tumor in the same breast or chest wall

local therapy: when only the breast is treated for breast cancer (surgery and/or radiation therapy is considered local therapy)

lumpectomy: a nickname for a breast conservation surgery that removes the lump (tumor) but conserves the breast; often combined with axillary dissection and external radiation therapy; lumpectomy at one time simply referred to removing a lump for biopsy, but this term is being discarded

lymph nodes: located under the arms, around the neck, and around the groin area, these act like little POW camps that hold and "interrogate" foreign invaders; they swell when they're active but are also common sites for cancer that has spread; enlarged lymph nodes should be brought to the attention of your doctor

lymphedema (arm edema): a condition in which the arm swells, caused by an axillary dissection

malignant: not benign and therefore cancerous, as in malignant tumor or malignancy

mammogram: a breast X ray requiring the breast to be compressed between two metal plates; mammograms are used as a method of routine screening for breast cancer in healthy women as well as a diagnostic tool to investigate women of any age with suspicious symptoms

mammography guidelines: guidelines that refer to the ideal age when routine breast screening should begin and at which intervals (annually, every two years, etc.); guidelines currently conflict—experts can't agree on whether routine breast screening should begin at age forty or fifty

manual breast exam: when your doctor examines your breast by carefully feeling it for lumps and changes; should be done as part of your annual physical

mastectomy: surgical removal of the breast; there are many different kinds of mastectomy procedures; see also wide lumpectomy and lumpectomy

menarche: a woman's first menstrual period; the average age of menarche in North America is 12.8 years old, and 17 years old in China

menopause: when the ovaries stop making estrogen

metastasis: a cancer that invades other tissue or spreads

metastatic disease (distant or systemic recurrence): a cancer that has spread to other organs; breast cancer usually spreads to bones or lungs, which may cause a variety of symptoms

modifiable risk: a risk that can be reduced, prevented, or altered through changing behavior, such as quitting smoking or dieting

narcotic (strong opioid): a powerful prescription drug used to control pain; narcotics used for severe pain control are generally not addictive; most narcotics used in advanced cancer treatment are morphine preparations and hydromorphine

needle biopsy: a simple in-office procedure in which a long needle is used to suck out cells and/or fluid from a lump for further investigation

node-negative: cancer that has not spread to the lymph nodes

node-positive: cancer that has spread to the lymph nodes

non-lactational mastitis: a bacterial breast infection of the breast in a woman who is not breastfeeding

non-narcotic: a painkiller that is not a narcotic, and hence often an over-the-counter medication that is not as potent; A.S.A., acetaminophen, and NSAIDs are all non-narcotics

nonylphenol: an ingredient in common plastics, found in detergents, toiletries, cosmetics, etc.

NSAID: acronym for non-steroidal anti-inflammatory drugs; a class of drugs used for relieving pain, such as ibuprofen; should be avoided prior to surgery

oncogenes: dormant genes that absorb various external "hits" until they switch on and tell cells to mutate

oncologist: cancer specialist; radiation oncologists specialize in radiation therapy for cancer patients, while medical oncologists specialize in chemotherapy for cancer patients

one-in-eight: lifetime risk of getting breast cancer if you live to age ninety-five

one-in-nine: lifetime risk of getting breast cancer if you live to age eighty-five; 1 in 9 is also the name of a breast cancer activist organization out of Long Island

oral contraceptives: birth control pills; available as combination oral contraceptives (with estrogen and progestin) or as a progestin-only pill, also known as the mini-pill

organochlorine: what you get when you take natural chlorine, found in ordinary salt, and link it up with organic materials

osteoporosis: bone loss; aggravated by estrogen loss after menopause

oxytocin: a hormone that stimulates the milk glands to secrete milk when breast-feeding and stimulates the uterus to contract, triggered by a baby or lover suckling the breast; oxytocin also makes the uterus contract during labor

palliative care: symptom relief and pain and symptom management; anyone who wants to feel free of symptoms is a palliative care patient

pathologist: a doctor who specializes in examining tissue and/or cells under a microscope; this doctor generates a pathology report (the "path report")

PCBs: abbreviation for polychlorinated biphenyls; a group of about two hundred toxic compounds mostly used for paints, inks, electrical equipment, and hydraulic fluids; these compounds are harmful to the environment and are now under stringent control by most governments

phytoestrogens: a source of natural estrogen from plants

postmenopausal breast cancer: breast cancer that develops after menopause

ppb: short for parts per billion

premenopausal breast cancer: breast cancer that develops before menopause

progestin: synthetically produced progesterone; a female hormone produced by the egg

prolactin: the hormone responsible for breast milk production, which can be inhibited by high levels of estrogen

prophylactic surgery: preventive surgery; prophylactic mastectomy is often recommended to women who come from a high-risk family

prosthesis: a false breast used after a mastectomy procedure; many women find that a prosthesis is a satisfying alternative to breast reconstruction

prn: means as needed in pharmacyspeak

radiation therapy: treatment that involves high-energy X rays or gamma rays to penetrate the skin

reconstruction surgery: surgery that follows a mastectomy procedure, which uses either your own tissue or implants to reconstruct your breast; many women have reconstructive surgery at the same time as a mastectomy

regional recurrence: a recurrence of the cancer in the axillary lymph nodes

relative risk: compares risk in situation A with risk in situation B (which is usually a standard or constant, such as a no-risk factor)

risk counseling: having family history, lifestyle, and genetic predispositions analyzed by an expert in breast cancer risk; most experts have a background in genetic counseling and charge roughly U.S. $350 as of 1996

saline: salt water; used instead of silicone gel as an alternate filler for breast implants

saturated fat: found in chocolate and tropical oils; this type of fat is solid at room temperature and stimulates the body to make cholesterol; worse than foods naturally high in cholesterol

secretory gland: a gland that secretes fluids, such as the breast

silicone: a synthetic jelly-like plastic material used to make breast implants; preferred because its texture closely approximates the texture of human breast tissue

staging: breast cancer can be diagnosed anywhere from stages 0 to 4; the staging refers to the size of the tumor as well as where the cancer has spread

statistically significant: when the probability is less than one in twenty of something being found *by chance*, it's said to be statistically significant

surgical menopause: menopause that results from medical treatment; most women who undergo chemotherapy prior to natural menopause will experience surgical menopause; estrogen loss symptoms are often more pronounced in this case

systemic therapy: treating the whole body, not just the breast; chemotherapy and hormone therapy are systemic therapies

tamoxifen: an anti-estrogen drug used in hormone therapy

therapeutic abortion: surgical termination of a pregnancy

TNM: acronym for tumor, node, metastasis; a classification method with a logical numbering system that doctors use to determine the stage of a cancer

trans-fatty acids: found in margarine or shortening, these have been linked to cardiovascular disease; they are made from the process of hydrogenation, which solidifies various oils

tumor: from the Latin *tumere*, which means to swell; this is a clump of cells that is growing and reproducing, forming a lump of some sort

white blood cells (WBC): cells made inside the bone marrow; these are important for your immune system; chemotherapy may lower your white blood cell count, causing you to be more vulnerable to infections

wide lumpectomy (wide excision): when a tumor and some normal breast tissue are removed, leaving the breast and surrounding lymph nodes intact; also known as partial mastectomy, quandrantectomy, and segmental mastectomy; *all* labels refer to this one procedure.

WHO: acronym for World Health Organization

Note: This list is not exhaustive. I've identified key words that are often misused, misunderstood, or usually not explained when dealing with breast cancer risk, detection, and treatment. All these words or terms are fully explained within the text of this book, as well. These are not literal dictionary definitions, but rather definitions created solely for the context of this book. Any resemblance to definitions found in other glossaries or dictionaries is purely coincidental.

BIBLIOGRAPHY

Background articles and general texts, tapes, and books

"Importance of Breast Health Activism." *Women's Wear Daily,* 31 August 1994, S14.

"The Politics of Breast Cancer." *Ms,* May/June 1993. Contains several articles on breast cancer.

"University of Pittsburgh and Allegheny Agreement Announced." *Cancer Biotechnology Weekly* (13 February 1995): 4.

Holman, Dawn, and Joy McDiarmid, producers. *Voices in the Night: A Cancer Companion, Diagnosis,* Winnipeg: Voices in the Night, Inc., 1993. Audiocassette.

Holman, Dawn, and Joy McDiarmid, producers. *Voices in the Night: A Cancer Companion, Early Breast Cancer Series,* Winnipeg: Voices in the Night, Inc., 1995. Audiocassette.

Holman, Dawn, and Joy McDiarmid, producers. *Voices in the Night: A Cancer Companion, Questions and Choices,* Winnipeg: Voices in the Night, Inc., 1994. Audiocassette.

Arsenault, Gillian. "Breast Cancer Epidemiology." Unpublished report, 1996.

Ayanian, John Z., Betsy A. Kohler, Toshi Abe, and Arnold M. Epstein. "The Relation between Health Insurance Coverage and Clinical Outcomes among Women with Breast Cancer." *New England Journal of Medicine.* 329, no. 5 (1993): 326–331.

Batt, Sharon. *Patient No More: The Politics of Breast Cancer.* Charlottetown, Penn.: gynergy books, 1994.

Burlington Breast Cancer Support Services, Inc. *What You Need to Know about Breast Cancer.* Burlington, Ont.: Burlington Breast Cancer Support Services, 1993.

Casciato, Dennis, and Barry B. Lowitz, eds. *Manual of Clinical Oncology,* 2nd ed., Boston: Little Brown, 1988.

Dolinger, Malin, Ernest H. Rosenbaum, and Greg Cable. *Everyone's Guide to Cancer Therapy.* Toronto, Ont.: Somerville House, 1995.

Drum, David. *Making The Chemotherapy Decision.* Los Angeles: Lowell House, 1996.

Engle, June. *The Complete Breast Book.* Toronto, Ont.: Key Porter Books, 1996.

Ferraro, Susan. "The Anguished Politics of Breast Bancer." *The New York Times Magazine,* 15 August 1993, 24.

Henderson, Craig I. "Paradigmatic Shifts in the Management of Breast Cancer." *New England Journal of Medicine* 332, no. 14 (April 1995): 951—952.

Hoy, Claire. *The Truth about Breast Cancer.* Toronto, Ont.: Stoddart Publishing, 1995.

Love, Susan, and Karen Lindsey, *Dr. Susan Love's Breast Book,* 2nd ed. New York: Addison-Wesley, 1995.

Olivotto, Ivo, Karen Gelman, and Urve Kuusk. *Breast Cancer.* Vancouver, B.C.: Intelligent Patient Guide, 1995.

Olmsted, Marcy. "A Doctor's Story." *Mirabella,* August 1993, 129—134.

CHAPTER 1 *(Who Gets Breast Cancer, and Why?)*

"Advocates Cite Cancer Rates in Calling for Pesticide Curbs." *The New York Times,* 18 February 1994, p. 6.

Greenpeace. *Body of Evidence: The Effects of Chlorine on Human Health.* Washington, D.C.: Greenpeace, 1994.

"Corporate Breast Cancer Education and Detection Fund Established." *Cancer Researcher Weekly* (7 February 1994): 10.

"EPA to Study Safety of an Insecticide." *The New York Times,* 24 October 1993, p. 10.

"Mortality Declines for Caucasian Women." *Cancer Biotechnology Weekly* (13 February 1995): 7.

"Passive Smoking, Other Factors, and Breast Cancer in Young Women." *Nutrition Research Newsletter* 13 (September 1994): 100.

Canadian Broadcasting Corporation. *Sex under Siege.* Documentary. 1994.

World Wildlife Fund Canada. "Toxics That Tamper with Hormones." *Eagles Eye.* (Summer 1995).

Anstett, Patricia. "Breast-Feeding Cuts Breast Cancer Risk, New Study Says." *Knight-Ridder/Tribune News Service,* 10 December 1993.

Associated Press. "High Levels of Saturated Fat Found to Promote Ovarian Cancer." *The New York Times,* 21 September 1994, p. C10.

Brody, Jane E. "Scientist at Work: Bruce N. Ames; Strong Views on Origins of Cancer. *The New York Times,* 5 July 1994, p. C1.

Chilvers, Clair. "Oral Contraceptives and Cancer." *The Lancet* 344 (19 November 1994): 1378.

Cotton, Paul. "Environmental Estrogenic Agents Area of Concern." *JAMA* 271 (9 February 1994): 414, 416.

Davis, D. L., et al. "Medical Hypothesis: Xenoestrogens as Preventable Causes of Breast Cancer." *Environmental Health Perspectives* 101 (1993): 372–377.

Dawson, P. J., et al. "MCF10AT: A Model for the Evolution of Breast Cancer from Proliferative Breast Disease." *American Journal of Pathology* 148 (January 1996): 313–319.

DeMarco, Carolyn. "Military Research: Endometriosis and Environmental Toxins Linked?" *Wellness MD* 4 (March/April 1994): 23

DeMarco, Carolyn. "Preserving Our Environment: Breast Cancer and the Environment." *Health Naturally* (October/November 1995): 26–30.

Dunn, Bruce. "The Israeli Breast Cancer Anomaly." *abreast* 1 (Winter 95–96): 5.

Epstein, Samuel S. "Pesticides Pose a Lifelong Threat." *The New York Times,* 29 August 1994, p. 14.

Epstein, Samuel S. "So You Consider Hair Dye Safe?" *The New York Times,* 16 February 1994, p. 20.

Fackelmann, K. A. "Do Abortions Heighten Breast Cancer Risk?" *Science News* 146 (5 November 1994): 294.

Gammon, J. E. Bertin, and M. B. Terry. "Abortion and the Risk of Breast Cancer. Is There a Believable Association?" *JAMA* 275 (24–31 January 1996): 321–322.

Gillis, Anna Maria. "Wildlife Indicators Worrying." *Bioscience* 44 (May 1994): 296–298.

Gills, Anna Maria. Research Update: From the Washington, D.C., Meeting on Estrogens in the Environment: Global Health Implications. *Bioscience* 44, no. 5: 296–298.

Highfield, Roger. "Gender-Bending Chemicals May Cause Cancers." *Daily Telegraph,* London, 26 July 1995, p. 4.

Harvey, Robin. "Bras and Breast Cancer." *The Toronto Star,* 18 March 1996.

Hodges, John. "Sperm—Down for the Count?" *Wellness MD* 3 (July/August 1993): 10.

Horsman, Doug. "Hereditary Cancer Testing and Counselling in BC." *abreast* 1 (Winter 95–96): 4–8.

Howe, Geoffrey, R. "Dietary Fat and Breast Cancer Risks." *Cancer Supplement* 74 (1 August 1994).

Hunter, David J., et al. "A Prospective Study of the Intake of Vitamins C, E, and A and the Risk of Breast Cancer." *New England Journal of Medicine* 329 (22 July 1993): 234–240.

Jackson, Phillip. "Grave Thoughts." *Wellness MD* 3 (July/August 1993): 19–21.

Johnson, Jeff. "Will Our Stolen Future Be Another Silent Spring?" *Environmental Science & Technology News* 30. (1996): 168–170.

Kelsey, Jennifer L., and Esther M. John. "Lactation and the Risk of Breast Cancer." *New England Journal of Medicine* 330 (13 January 1994): 136–137.

LeBlanc, Gerald A. "Are Environmental Sentinels Signaling?" *Environmental Health Perspectives* 103 (October 1995).

Li, D., M. Wang, K. Dhingra, and W. N. Hittelman. "Aromatic DNA Adducts in Adjacent Tissues of Breast Cancer Patients: Clues to Breast Cancer Etiology." *Cancer Res.* 56 (15 January 1996): 287–293.

Linton, Marilyn. "Offering Novel Thoughts on Breast Cancer. "*The Sunday Sun,* 4 February 1996, p. 52. Column based on interview with Canadian Breast Cancer chairman Dr. Steve Narod.

Munson, Marty. "Cancer Cruncher: Workouts May Be Your Breast Protection." *Prevention* 47 (January 1995): 27.

Newcomb, P. A., et al. "Pregnancy Termination in Relation to Risk of Breast Cancer." *JAMA* 275 (24–31 January 1996): 283–287.

Newcomb, Polly A., et al. "Lactation and a Reduced Risk of Premenopausal Breast Cancer." *New England Journal of Medicine* 330 (13 January 1994): 81–87.

Newschaffer, C. J., et al. "The Effect of Age and Comorbidity in the Treatment of

Elderly Women with Nonmetastatic Breast Cancer." *Archives of Internal Medicine* 156 (8 January 1996): 85–90.

Ramlow, J. M., G. W. Olsen, and G. G. Bond. "Environment Health Link Calls for Study." *Environmental Protection* 5 (1994): 63–68.

Raloff, Janet. "Menstrual Cycles May Affect Cancer Risk." *Science News* 147 (7 January 1995): 7.

Raloff, Janet. "Obesity, Diet Linked to Breast Cancer." *Science News* 147 (21 January 1995): 39.

Raloff, Janet. "Ecocancers." *Science News* 144 (3 July 1993): 10–13.

Raloff, J. A. "Plastics May Shed Chemical Estrogens." *Science News* 144 (3 July 1993): 12.

Rather, John. "L. I. Is Pressuring Albany to Check Perils of Pesticides." *The New York Times,* 27 February 1994, p. 1 (Section 13LI).

Reaney, Patricia. "Report Probes Chemical Link to Disappearing Sperm." Reuters News Service, London, 25 July 1995.

Rosenberg, L., et al. "Case-Control Study of Oral Contraceptive Use and Risk of Breast Cancer." *American Journal of Epidemiology* 143 (1 January 1996): 25–37.

Sachs, Jessica Snyder. "Hidden Dangers in Your Food and Water." *McCalls* 121, August 1994, 40.

Schemo, Diana Jean. "L. I. Breast Cancer Is Possibly Linked to Chemical Sites." *The New York Times,* 13 April 1994, p. 1.

Shore, Laurence S., Michael Gurevitz, and Mordechai Shemesh. "Estrogen As an Environmental Pollutant." *Bulletin of Environmental Contamination and Toxicology* 51 (September 1993): 361–366.

Soto, Ana M., et al. "*p*-Nonyl-Phenol: An Estrogenic Xenobiotic Released from Modified Polystyrene." *Environmental Health Perspectives* 92 (1991): 167–173.

Soto, Ana M., Kerrie L. Chung, and Carlos Sonnenschein. "The Pesticides Endosulfan, Toxaphene, and Dieldrin Have Estrogenic Effects on Human Estrogen-Sensitive Cells." *Environmental Health Perspectives* 102 (February 1994).

Steinberg, W. M. "Menopause and Breast Cancer." *Patient Care* (May 1993): 8.

Stevens, William K. "Pesticides May Leave Legacy of Hormonal Chaos." *The New York Times,* 23 August 1994, p. C1 (Science section).

Thornton, Joe. "Chlorine, Human Health and the Environment: The Breast Cancer Warning." Washington, D.C.: Greenpeace, 1993.

CHAPTER 2 (Is It Cancer?)

"Evaluation of a Breast Mass." *NEJM* 328 (1993): 810–812.

Bass, Brenda, Diane Pross, and Peter Bell. "Recruitment for Breast Screening in a Rural Practice: Trial of a Physician's Letter of Invitation." *Canadian Family Physician* 40 (October 1994): 1730–1739.

Elmore Joann G., et al. "Variability in Radiologists Interpretations of Mammograms." *New England Journal of Medicine* 331 (1 December 1994): 1493–1499.

Feig, S. A. "Estimation of Currently Attainable Benefit from Mammographic Screening of Women Aged 40–49 Years." *Cancer* 75 no. 1186 (1995): 2412–2419.

Kopans, D. B. "Mammography Screening for Breast Cancer." *Cancer* 72 no. 439 (1993): 1809–1812.

Long, Patricia. "More Than 90 Percent of Women Diagnosed with Early Breast Cancer Survive." *Health Magazine*, 1995, Document mpl395c.

Hammond, Jo-Anne, Marie Smithers, and Moira Stewart. "Female Patients Attitudes to Mammography Screening." *Canadian Family Physician* 40 (March 1994): 451–455.

Kopans, Daniel B. "The Accuracy of Mammographic Interpretation." *New England Journal of Medicine* 331 (1 December 1994): 1521–1522.

Kotwall, Cyrus, and Lavina Lickley. "On the Alert for Breast lumps." *Patient Care* (April 1993): 15–30.

Lindfors, K. K., Rosenquist, J. "The Cost-Effectiveness of Mammographic Screening Strategies." *JAMA* 274, no. 1482 (1995): 881–884.

Lubin, F. "A Case-Control Study of Caffeine and Methylxanthines in Benign Breast Disease." *JAMA* no. 196 (1985): 2388–2392.

Lurie, Nicole, Jonathan Slater, and Paul McGovern. "Preventive Care for Women: Does the Sex of the Physician Matter?" *New England Journal of Medicine* no. 7 (12 August 1993): 478.

Weber, Barbara L. "Clinical Implications of Basic Research: Susceptibility genes for Breast Cancer." *New England Journal of Medicine* 331 (1 December 1994): 1523–1524.

Willett, Walter C., and David J. Hunter. "Prospective Studies of Diet and Breast Cancer." *Cancer Supplement* 74 (August 1, 1994).

CHAPTER 3 *(When They Say It's Malignant)*

Ductal Carcinoma In Situ of the Breast: Understanding the Misunderstood Stepchild. *JAMA* 275 (27 March 1996): 948–949.

Casciato, Dennis, and Barry B. Lowitz, eds. *Manual of Clinical Oncology,* 2nd ed. Boston: Little Brown, 1988.

Dolinger, Malin, Ernest H. Rosenbaum, and Greg Cable. *Everyone's Guide to Cancer Therapy.* Toronto: Somerville House, 1995.

Drexler, Madeline. "It's Almost Cancer: What Now?" McCalls, March 1996.

Ernster, Virginia L., et al. "Incidence of and Treatment for Ductal Carcinoma In Situ of the Breast." *JAMA 275* (27 March 1996): 913–918.

Snyderman, Nancy. "Breast Cancer Therapies: One Size Does Not Fit All." *Good Housekeeping,* April 1996.

CHAPTER 4 *(Life after Surgery)*

Adriamycin RDF Product Monograph. Pharmacia, 1995.

Adrucil Product Monograph. Pharmacia, 1995.

Benedet, Rosalind Delores. *Healing: A Woman's Guide to Recover after Mastectomy.* San Francisco: R. Benedet Publishing, 1993.

Casciato, Dennis, and Barry B. Lowitz, ed., *Manual of Clinical Oncology,* 2nd ed. Boston: Little Brown, 1988.

Cukier, Daniel. *Ray of Hope: Coping with Radiation Therapy.* Los Angeles: Lowell House, 1994.

Cytotoxan Product Monograph. Bristol, 1995.

Dolinger, Malin, Ernest H. Rosenbaum, and Greg Cable. *Everyone's Guide to Cancer Therapy.* Toronto, Ont.: Somerville House, 1995.

Drum, David. *Making the Chemotherapy Decision.* Los Angeles: Lowell House, 1996.

Howell A. Mackintosh, et al. "The Definition of the No-Change Category in Patients Treated with Endocrine Therapy and Chemotherapy for Advanced Carcinoma of the Breast." *European Journal of Clinical Oncology* 24 (1988): 1567–1572.

Mathieson, Cynthia M. "Invitations to Listen: Cancer Talk, Body Talk." *The Canadian Journal of OB/Gyn & Women's Health Care* 6 no. 7 (1994): 716–722.

Methotrexate Product Monograph. Liderle, 1995.

Nolvadex (Tamoxifen Citrate) Product Monograph. Zeneca, 1995.

Oncovin Product Monograph. Lilly, 1995.

Pharmorubicin RDF (Eprirubicin HCI) Product Monograph. Pharmacia, 1995.

Plourde, P. V., and Dowsett M. Dyroff, et al. "Arimidex: A New Oral Once-a-Day Aromatase Inhibitor." *Journal of Biochemical Biology* 53 (1995): 175–179.

Plourde, P. V., M. Dyroff, and M. Dukes. "Arimidex: A Potent and Selective Fourth-Generation Aromatase Inhibitor." *Breast Cancer Rest Treat.* 30 (1994): 103–111.

Robertson J. F. R., et al. "Factors Predicting the Response of Patients with Advanced Breast Cancer to Endocrine Therapy." *European Journal of Clinical Oncology* 23 (1989): 469–475.

CHAPTER 5 (*Reconstruction and Alternatives*)

"Breast Implants on Trial." *Frontline.* Documentary. *27* February 1996.

Anderson, Pauline. "Another Group Says No Evidence for Link between Silicone and Auto-immunity." *Medical Post.* May 1996.

Rees, Alan M. "Breast implants: Everything You Need to Know." In *The Consumer Health Information Source Book,* 4th ed. Oryx Press, 1994, p. 139. (Review of *Breast implants: Everything You Need to Know,* Nancy Bruning, Alameda, CA: Hunter House, 1992.)

Richardson, Sarah. "Implant Innocence? Health Hazards of Breast Implants." *Discover* 16 (January 1995): 73.

Romanelli, James N. "More on Breast Implants and Connective-Tissue Diseases." *New England Journal of Medicine* 332 (11 May 1995): 1306.

Solomon, Gary, Luis Espinoza, and Stuart Silverman. "Breast Implants and Connective-Tissue Diseases." *New England Journal of Medicine* 331 (3 November 1994): 1231.

CHAPTER 6 (*Friends and Lovers*)

Block, Jean Libman. "My Husband and I Have Breast Cancer." *Good Housekeeping.* February 1995, 46.

Clash, James M. "What Men Can Do to Help." *Forbes* 153, 20 June 1994, 122.

McGough, Michael. "When It's Your Wife: What Does Mastectomy Mean to a Husband?" *American Health* 12 (September 1993): 44.

CHAPTER 7 *(All about Complementary Medicine)*

Bagley, Gordon. "Magic or Medicine: In Praise of the Healing Touch." *Wellness MD* 4 (January/February 1994): 31–38.

Chisholm, Patricia. "Healers or Quacks? The Controversy over Unconventional Treatments." *Macleans*, 25 September 1995, 34–42.

Harvey, Rosin. "To Do No Harm: Healers and Heretics." *The Toronto Star*, 27 January 1996, p. L1.

Griffin, Katherine. "Alternative Care: Finally Some Coverage." *Health Magazine*, 1995, Document mkgo95a.

Long, Patricia. "Herbal Remedies Really Can Fight Off Colds, Headaches and Other Ills—If You Know How to Use Them Safely." *Health Magazine*, 1995, Document mpl595h.

Weiss, Rick. "The FDA may soon concede that billions of Chinese were right all along: Acupuncture works." *Health Magazine*, 1995, Document mrwl95a.

CHAPTER 8 *(The Second Time Around)*

"New Genetic Markers May Help Predict Whether Cancer Will Return." *Cancer Researcher Weekly* (25 April 1994): 17.

"Significance of Family History in Treatment of Breast Cancer." *American Family Physician* 50 (December 1994): 1802. Article adapted from the *Journal of the American College of Surgeons*, July 1994.

"What Are the Chances of Getting Recurrent Breast Cancer." *Cancer Weekly* (11 January 1993): 4.

Mraz, Sharon J. Towner. "When Relapse Occurs: One Woman's Perspective." *BMT Newsletter* (May 1994).

Munson, Marty. "Slim Breast-Cancer Risks: Staying Slender Could Hold Off a Cancer Rerun." *Prevention* 46 (July 1994): 30.

CHAPTER 9 *(Palliative Care)*

Health and Welfare Canada, Expert Advisory Committee on the management of severe chronic pain in cancer patients. *Cancer Pain.* [Ottawa]: Health and Welfare Canada, 1984.

Casciato, Dennis, and Barry B. Lowitz, eds. *Manual of Clinical Oncology*, 2nd ed. Boston: Little Brown, 1988.

Howarth, Gillian, and Kathleen Baba Willison. "Preventing Crises in Palliative Care in the Home." *Canadian Family Physician* 41 (March 1995): 439–445.

Jones, Charmaine M., and Jessica Pegis. *The Palliative Patient: Principles of Treatment.* Markham, Ont.: Knoll Pharma Inc., 1994.

Librach, S. Lawrence. *The Pain Manual: Principles and Issues in Cancer Pain Management.* Published in association with the Canadian Cancer Society, 1990.

MacDonald, Neil. "Palliative Care in Pain Treatment." *Cancer Pain: IASP refresher course syllabus,* 1994.

McWhinney, Ian R., and M. A. Stewart. "Home Care of Dying Patients." *Canadian Family Physician* 40 (February 1994): 240–246.

Pain Management Newsletter. Knoll Pharma Inc. June 1994 Supplement.

Pain Management Newsletter. Knoll Pharma Inc. Vol. 8, no. 1 (April 1995).

Pain Management Newsletter. Knoll Pharma Inc. Vol. 8, no. 2 (August 1995).

Thackeray, B. D. "Practice Observed: Some Haven't Got time for the Pain." *Wellness MD* 4 (March/April 1994): 35–37.

CHAPTER 10 *(What about Prevention?)*

"Cancer Center Studies Link between Dietary Fat and Breast Cancer." *Cancer Researcher Weekly* (28 February 1994): 8.

"Cancer-Cell Detection Methods—Breast Cancer Vaccine Development." *Cancer Biotechnology Weekly* (30 January 1995): 6.

Cornell University. "Estrogens in Vegetables May Reduce Hot Flashes and Breast Cancer Risk, Cornell University Nutritionist Says." Press Release, Cornell University. 17 February 1994.

"Diet and Breast Cancer." *Nutrition Research Newsletter* 13 (September 1994): 101. Adapted from *Archives Internal Medicine,* 22 August 1994, and *British Journal of Cancer,* September 1994.

"Fruits, Vegetables Shield against Breast Cancer." *Better Nutrition for Today's Living* 56, July 1994, 18.

"Garlic Acts as an Anti-carcinogen in Breast Cancer." *Cancer Researcher Weekly* (17 January 1994): 3.

"Olive Oil and Breast Cancer: How Strong a Connection?" *The University of California, Berkeley Wellness Letter* 11 (April 1995).

Allison, Malorye. "Breast Cancer: Moving toward Prevention." *Harvard Health Letter* 17 (August 1992): 4–6.

Bagley, Gordon. "Self-help and Self-care: Patient Profiles Are Changing—Are You Ready?" *Wellness MD* 2 (November/December 1992).

Behen, Madonna. "The New Breast Cancer Test: The Discovery of the Breast Cancer Gene Is a Medical Milestone ... What You Need to Know." *Good Housekeeping*, April 1996.

Bagley, Gordon. "Wellness and Medicine: Spare Us All That New Age Jazz." *Wellness MD* 2 (November/December 1992).

DeMarco, Carolyn. "Keys to the Highway." *Wellness MD* 3 (November/December 1993).

DeMarco, Carolyn. "The Great Mammogram Debate: Are We Spending Millions to Do Naught for Ought?" *Wellness MD* 3 (January/February 1993).

Kotz, Deborah. "The Mighty Mammogram: What It Can and Can't Do." *Weight Watchers Magazine* 27, May 1994, 34.

Kushi, Michio. *The Cancer Prevention Guide*. New York: St. Martins Press, 1993.

Liebman, Bonnie. "Breast Cancer." *Nutrition Action Health Letter*. January/February 1996.

Ontario Task Force on the Primary Prevention of Cancer. *Recommendations for the Primary Prevention of Cancer: Report of the Ontario Task Force on the Primary Prevention of Cancer*. Toronto, Ont.: March 1995. Presented to the Ontario Ministry of Health.

Popcorn, Faith. *The Popcorn Report*. New York: Doubleday, 1991.

Rennie, Susan. "Breast Cancer Prevention: Diet vs. Drugs." *Ms.*, May/June 1993, 38–57.

Willett, Walter C., and David J. Hunter. "Prospective Studies of Diet and Breast Cancer." *Cancer Supplement* 74 (1 August 1994).

*Additional resources for this edition:**

Bankhead, Charles. "NSAID Use Linked to Reduction in CA Risk." *Family Practice* (12 February 1996): 28.

Bernstein, Leslie, and Jennifer L. Kelsey. "Epidemiology and Prevention of Breast Cancer." Department of Health Research and Policy, Stanford University, and Department of Preventive Medicine, University of Southern California (1996): 47-67.

*In light of the subject matter, this book has been updated substantially since it was introduced in 1996. Dozens of new sources were used for this softcover edition. An updated bibliography may be obtained by request from the publisher: Lowell House, 2020 Avenue of the Stars, Suite 300, Los Angeles, CA 90067; fax 310-552-7573.

"Breast Cancer and Abortion." *New Woman* (April 1997): 99.

Brind, Joel, Vernon M. Chinchilli, Walter B. Severs, and Joan Summy-Long. "Induced Abortion as an Independent Risk Factor for Breast Cancer." Department of Natural Sciences, City University of New York, and Center for Biostatistics and Epidemiology and Department of Pharmacology, Pennsylvania State University (1996).

"Chemical in Green Tea Stops Tumors, Study Says." *Reuters* (5 June 1997).

Colborn, Theo, John Peterson Myers, Dianne Dumanoski. *Our Stolen Future.* New York: Dutton, 1996.

"Drug-Resistant Cancer Revealed." *Journal of Biological Chemistry* (273; 1997): 1-6.

"Exercise and Breast Cancer—Time to Get Moving?" *New England Journal of Medicine* 336 (1 May 1997).

Gofman, John W. *Preventing Breast Cancer: The Story of a Major, Proven, Preventable Cause of This Disease.* San Francisco: CNR Book Division, Committee for Nuclear Responsibility, 1995.

International Joint Commission. *Eighth Biennial Report on Great Lakes Water Quality, Under the Great Lakes Water Quality Agreement of 1978 to the Governments of the United States and Canada and the State and Provincial Governments of the Great Lakes Basin.* (1996)

Plotkin, David. "Good News and Bad News about Breast Cancer." *The Atlantic Monthly* (June 1996): 53-82.

Robson, Barbara. "Conferences Point to Growing Concern about Possible Links Between Breast Cancer, Environment." *Canadian Medical Association Journal* 8 (15 April 1996): 1254.

Steingraber, Sandra. *Living Downstream: An Ecologist Looks at Cancer and the Environment.* New York: Addison-Wesley: 1997.

"Three Types of Breast Cancer?" *Reuters,* from *The New York Times* (1 April 1997).

"Tulane Researcher Claims Antibodies Found to Silicone in Breast Implants." *The Associated Press* (14 February 1997).

"breastcancer.com"

WHERE TO GO FOR MORE INFORMATION

Note: This list was compiled from dozens of sources. Because of the volatile nature of many health and non-profit organizations, some of the addresses and phone numbers below may have changed since this list was compiled. American and Canadian resources are listed separately. Canadians looking for specific topics should review the United States list as well. Canadian calls are welcomed by American organizations, and vice versa. Many of these organizations will have email addresses, which, due to the enormous length of the lists, are not generally provided at this time. As this book becomes updated, and more organizations go online, email addresses will be incorporated. Increasingly, though, lists like this one—at the back of a paper book—are going the way of the dinosaur. Many more resources can be found through the Internet (see Breast Cancer Online at the end of this list).

UNITED STATES

GENERAL INFORMATION

American Association for Cancer
Education
   MD Anderson Cancer Center
   151 Holcombe Boulevard
   Houston, TX 77030
   (713) 792-3020
   Fax (713) 792-0807

American Cancer Society (ACS)
   1599 Clifton Road NE
   Atlanta, GA 30329
   1-800-ACS-2345
   (404) 320-3333
   Fax (404) 325-0230

Breast Cancer Advisory Center (BCAC)
P.O. Box 224
Kensington, MD 20895
Fax (301) 949-1132

Cancer Care
1180 Avenue of the Americas
New York, NY 10036
(212) 221-3300

Cancer Control Society (CCS)
2043 N. Berendo Street
Los Angeles, CA 90027
(213) 663-7801

Cancer Information Service
Office of Cancer Information
NCI/NIH, Building 31, 10A07
9000 Rockville Pike
Bethesda, MD 20892
1-800-4-CANCER
Fax (301) 402-0555

Candelighters Childhood Cancer
Foundation
7910 Woodmont Avenue, Suite 460
Bethesda, MD 20814-3015
1-800-366-2223
Fax (301) 718-2686

CANHELP
3111 Paradise Bay Road
Port Ludlow, WA 98365-9771
(206) 437-2291

The Chemotherapy Foundation, Inc.
183 Madison Avenue
New York, NY 10016
(212) 213-9292

The Komen Alliance
The Susan G. Komen Foundation
Occidental Tower
5005 LBJ Freeway, Suite 370 LB74
Dallas, TX 75244
(214) 450-1777
1-800-IM-AWARE

National Alliance of Breast Cancer
Organizations (NABCO)
9 E. 37th Street, 10th Floor
New York, NY 10016
(212) 719-0154
Fax (212) 689-1213

National Breast Cancer Awareness
Month
P.O. Box 57424
Washington, D.C. 20036
(202) 785-0710

National Cancer Institute (NCI)
Office of Cancer Communications, NCI
Building 31, Room 10 A18
Bethesda, MD 20205
1-800-4-CANCER
(301) 496-5583

National Coalition for Cancer
Survivorship (NCCS)
1010 Wayne Avenue, 5th Floor
Silver Spring, MD 20910
(301) 650-8868
Fax (301) 565-9670

Patient Advocates for Advanced Cancer
Treatment
    1143 Parmelee NW
    Grand Rapids, MI 49504-3844
    (616) 453-1477
    Fax (616) 453-1846

Reach to Recovery
    c/o American Cancer Society
    (see above address under American
    Cancer Society)

The Rose Kushner Breast Cancer
Advisory Center
    P.O. Box 224
    Kensington, MD 20895
    (301) 949-2531

The Wellness Community
    2716 Ocean Park Boulevard,
    Suite 1040
    Santa Monica, CA 90405
    (310) 314-2555

Y-ME National Breast Cancer
Organization
    212 W. Van Buren Street
    Chicago, IL 60607
    (312) 986-8228 (24 hours)
    1-800-221-2141
    (9:00 A.M. to 5:00 P.M. CST)

AUDIO SUPPORT PROGRAMS

Voices in the Night: A Cancer Companion
    Box 24059
    1853 Grant Avenue
    Winnipeg, Manitoba, Canada R3N 2B1
    1-800-268-0009
    website:
    http://www.voicesinthenight.com

The Early Breast Cancer Series

This complete six-cassette, six-and-a-half
hour audio program is $49.95. Bound
transcripts are also available (if you do not
have sound capabilities) for the same cost,
or for an extra $20 with the cassettes.
Bulk orders of five or more are available at
a 20 to 40 percent discount (delivery to
one address, please).

Diagnosis

Done in the same style as the *Early
Breast Cancer Series*. This two-hour
cassette program is available for $19.95.
Bound transcripts are also available at the
same cost.

Questions and Choices

By the same producers, this program
helps you sort out all of your options
after a cancer diagnosis. This two-hour
twenty-minute program is available for
$19.95. Bound transcripts are also avail-
able at the same cost.

BREAST SPECIALISTS

American Society of Clinical Oncology
(ASCO)
  The American Board of Medical
  Specialists at 1-800-776-2378
  American College of Surgeons
  55 East Erie Street
  Chicago, IL 60611
  (312) 664-4050

American Society of Plastic and
  Reconstructive Surgeons
  1-800-635-0635

DATABASE SERVICES

Cancerfax
  NCI's Physician's Data Query (PDQ)
  (301) 402-5874

CANCERLIT
  1-800-950-2035

MEDLARS, MEDLINE
  1-800-272-4787

FINANCES AND INSURANCE

The Access Program
  10100 Santa Monica Boulevard,
  Suite 420
  Los Angeles, CA 90027
  1-800-235-6411
  (will convert life insurance into cash)

Affording Care National Center of
Financial information for Serious Illness
or Injury
  429 East 52nd Street, Suite 4G
  New York, NY 10022-6431
  (212) 371-4740

American Life Resources Corporation
  930 Washington Avenue, 4th Floor
  Miami, FL 31139
  1-800-633-0407

Cancer Centers
  11600 Nobel Street, Suite 201
  Rockville, MD 20852
  (301) 984-9496.

Cancer: Treatments Your Insurance
Should Cover (booklet)
  The Association of Community
  The National Insurance Consumer
  Helpline 1-800-942-4242.

Living Benefits, Inc.
  6110 Seagull Lane NE, Suite 108
  Albuquerque, NM 87109
  1-800-458-8790 or (505) 833-4799

National Insurance Consumer
Organization
  P.O. Box 15492
  Alexandria, VA 22309
  (703) 549-8050
  1-800-942-4242

HAIR LOSS

American Hair Loss Council
  1-800-274-8717

Buyer's Guide to Wigs and Hairpieces
  Ruth L. Weintraub
  420 Madison Avenue, Suite 406
  New York, NY 10017
  (212) 838-1333

Edith Imre Foundation for Loss of Hair
  30 West 57th Street
  New York, NY 10019
  (212) 757-8160

Soft Options
  6345 Galletta Drive
  Newark, CA 94560
  (510) 797-8188

Wig Hotline
  (212) 765-8397

Y-Me Prosthesis and Wig Bank
  1-800-221-2141

HOTLINES

American Cancer Society
  1-800-ACS-2345

AMC Cancer Research Center's Cancer
Information Line
  1-800-525-3777

Ask-A-Nurse
  1-800-535-1111

ASPRS
Plastic Surgery Information Service
  1-800-635-0635

Cancer Care Counseling Line
  1-800-813-HOPE

Cancer Care, Inc., and the National
Cancer Care Foundation
  1180 Avenue of the Americas
  New York, NY 10036
  (212) 211-3300

Cancer Helpline
  1-800-UMC-2215

FDA Breast Implant Hotline
  1-800-532-4440

Memorial Sloan-Kettering Cancer
Center
  1275 York Avenue
  New York, NY 10021
  1-800-525-2225
  (9:00 A.M. to 5:00 P.M., Monday to
  Friday)

National Cancer Institute
  1-800-4-CANCER

Women's Health Initiative
  1-800-54-WOMEN

LYMPHEDEMA

Breast Cancer Physical Therapy Center
  1905 Spruce Street
  Philadelphia, PA 19103

National Lymphedema Network and
Network Hotline
  2211 Post Street, Suite 404
  San Francisco, CA 94115
  1-800-541-3259

MAMMOGRAPHY GUIDELINES

1-800-358-9295
  (free booklet)

PALLIATIVE CARE

The National Hospice Organization in
  Arlington, VA
  1-800-658-8898
  1-800-331-1620

PESTICIDES

Pesticide Action Network North
America (PANNA)
  116 New Montgomery Street,
    Suite 810
  San Francisco, CA 94105
  (415) 541-9140
  Fax: (415) 541-9253
  Email: panna@igc.apc.org

PRESCRIPTIONS BY MAIL ORDER

American Preferred Prescription
  1-800-227-1195

BIO-LOGICS - THE R X RESOURCE
  1-800-850-4306

MEDI-EXPRESS R X
  1-800-873-9773

PROSTHESIS

Charming with Dignity
  112 West 34th Street, Suite 1617
  New York, NY 10120
  1-800-477-8188.

External Reconstruction Technology, Inc.
  4535 Benner Street
  Philadelphia, PA 19135
  (215) 333-8424

Ladies First Choice
  6465 Sunnyside Road SE
  Salem, OR 97306
  (503) 363-3940

Lady Grace Stores
  1-800-922-0504

My Secret
  41 West 86th Street
  New York, NY 10024
  (212) 877-8860

New Beginnings
  1556 Third Avenue, Room 603
  New York, NY 10128
  (212) 369-6630

Schwartz' Intimate Apparel
  108 Skokie Boulevard
  Wilmette, IL 60091
  (708) 251-1118

Underneath It All
444 East 75th Street
New York, NY 10021

PSYCHOSOCIAL SUPPORT
Wellness Community
310-314-2555

RECONSTRUCTION
American Society of Plastic and
Reconstructive Surgeons
444 East Algonquin Road
Arlington Heights, IL 60005
(312) 228-9900
1-800-635-0635

Command Trust Network
256 South Linden Drive
Beverly Hills, CA 90212
(310) 556-1738

Command Trust Network
The Breast Implant Information
Network
1-800-887-6828
Attorney Settlement information
(513) 651-9770

Plastic Surgery Information Service
Department of Communications
Executive Office 444
Last Algonquin Road
Arlington Heights, IL 60005

RISK COUNSELING
Risk Counseling and Research Centers
Strang Cancer Prevention Center
National High Risk Registry
428 East 72nd Street
New York, NY 10021
1-800-521-9356
(212) 794-4900

Women at Risk
Columbia-Presbyterian Medical
Center Breast Service
New York, NY 10032
(212) 305-9926

SCREENING
National Consortium of Breast Centers
c/o Barbara Rabinowitz, R.N., M.S.W.,
A.C.S.W.,
Comprehensive Breast Center
Robert Wood Johnson Medical School
One Robert Wood Johnson Place,
CN19
New Brunswick, NJ 08903-0019

SEX AND BREAST CANCER
The American Association of Sex
Educators, Counselors and Therapists
435 North Michigan Avenue, 1717
Chicago, IL 60611
(312) 644-0828

CANADA

NATIONAL

General

Alliance of Breast Cancer Survivors
P.O. Box 2035
20 Eglinton Avenue W
Toronto, ON M4R 1K8
(416) 487-9899
Fax (416) 487-0584

Breast Cancer Action
Billings Bridge Plaza
P.O. Box 39041
Ottawa, ON K1H1A1
(613) 736-5921
Fax (613) 736-8422

Breast Cancer Information Exchange
Project
Preventive Health Service Division
Health Canada
Jean Mance Building, Room 641
Tunney's Pasture
Ottawa, ON K1A 1B4
(613) 954-8668
Fax (613) 941-2633

Breast Implant Line of Canada
56 Touraine Avenue
North York, ON M3H1R2
(416) 636-6618

Canadian Breast Cancer Foundation
620 University Avenue, 9th Floor
Toronto, ON M5G 2C1
(416) 596-6773 or 1-800-387-9816

Canadian Breast Cancer Network
P.O. Box 39022
RPO Billings
Ottawa, ON K1H 1A1

Canadian Cancer Society
National Office
10 Alcorn Avenue, Suite 200
Toronto, ON M4V 3B1
(416) 961-7223
Fax (416) 961-4189

Canadian Cancer Society
Alberta/NWT
2424 4th Street SW, 2nd Floor
Calgary, AB T2S 2T4
(403) 228-4487

Cross Cancer Institute
11560 University Avenue
Edmonton, AB T6G1Z2
(403) 432-8763

Tom Baker Cancer Centre
1331 29th Street NW
Calgary, AB T2N 4N2
(403) 270-1700

Canadian Palliative Care Association
5 Blackburn Avenue
Ottawa, ON K1N 8A2
(613) 230-3354 or 1-800-668-2785
Fax (613-230-4376

Mission Air Transportation Network
   10 Alcorn Avenue, Suite 200
   Toronto, ON M4V 3Bl
   (416) 924-9333
   Fax (416) 924-5685
   (Nation-wide program to give cancer
   patients the use of available seats on
   corporate aircraft.)

The Neutropenia Support Association,
Inc.
   905 Corydon Avenue
   P.O. Box 243
   Winnipeg, MN R3M 3S7
   1-800-6-NEUTRO or 1-800-663-8876

Ontario Cancer Treatment and Research
Foundation
   620 University Avenue
   Toronto, ON M5G 2L7
   (416) 971-9800
   Fax (416) 971-6888

United Ostomy Association of
Canada, Inc.
   P.O. Box 46057
   College Park Post Office
   444 Yonge Street
   Toronto, ON M5B 2L8
   (416) 595-5452
   Fax (416) 595-9924

"Wellspring" (Support Group)
   The Coach House
   81 Wellesley Street E
   Toronto, ON M4Y 1H6
   (416) 961-1928
   Fax (416) 961-3721

Willow Breast Cancer Support and
Resource Center
   519 Jarvis Street, 2nd Floor
   Toronto, ON M4Y 1H7
   (416) 926-4537
   Fax (416) 926-6521

Audio Support Programs
See under United States for a description.

Hotlines
Cancer Information Service
   (Ontario only)
   1-800-263-6750

Consumer Health Information Service
   1-800-667-1999

Pesticides
Citizens for Alternatives to Pesticides
(CAP)
   20 Sunny Acres
   Baie d'Urfe, Québec H9X 3B6
   (514) 457-4347
   (514) 457-4840

Prosthesis Designer Swimwear
Linda Lundstom Ltd.
   33 Mallard Road
   Toronto, ON M3B 1S4
   416-391-2838.
   Call 1-800-66-LINDA for a current
   list of stores that carry her swimwear.

PROVINCIAL

Alberta

Alberta Cancer Board
  9707-110 Street, 6th Floor
  Edmonton, AB T5K 2L9
  (403) 782-3491
  (403) 585-8698
  (for AB, SK, MB, NWT)

Breast Cancer Info Link
  (Prairies/NWT)
  1331-29 Street NW
  Calgary, AB T2N 4N2
  (403) 670-2113
  Fax (403) 283-1651

British Columbia

B.C. Yukon Breast Cancer Information
Project
  565 West 10th Avenue
  Vancouver, BC V5Z 4J4
  (604) 872-4400
  Fax (604) 879-4533

Canadian Cancer Society British
  Columbia/Yukon
  565 West 10th Avenue
  Vancouver, BC V5Z 4J4
  (604) 872-4400

Cancer Control Agency of British
  Columbia
  600 West 10th Avenue
  Vancouver, BC V5Z 4E6
  (604) 877-6000

Cancer Information Service
  565 West 10th Avenue
  Vancouver, BC V5Z 4J4
  in Vancouver: (604) 879-2323
  outside Vancouver: 1-800-663-4242
  Fax (604) 879-9267

Victoria Cancer Clinic
  1900 Fort Street
  Victoria, BC V8R 1J8

Manitoba

Canadian Cancer Society
  193 Sherbrook Street
  Winnipeg, MB R3C 2B7
  (204) 774-7483

Manitoba Cancer Treatment and
Research Foundation
  100 Olivia Street
  Winnipeg, MB R3E 0V9
  (204) 787-2271

New Brunswick

Canadian Cancer Society
  P.O. Box 2089
  63 Union Street
  Saint John, NB E2L 3T5
  (506) 634-6272

Newfoundland and Labrador

Canadian Cancer Society
  P.O. Box 8921
  Chimo Building, 1st Floor
  St. John's, NF A1B 3R9
  (709) 753-6520

Newfoundland Cancer Clinic
Health Sciences Centre
   Prince Philip Drive
   St. John's, NF A1B 3V6
   (709) 737-6439

Newfoundland Cancer Treatment and
Research Foundation
   25 Kenmount Road
   St. John's, NF A1B 1W1

Nova Scotia

Canadian Cancer Society
   5826 South Street, Suite 1
   Halifax, NS B3H 1S6
   (902) 423-6183

Cancer Treatment and Research
Foundation of Nova Scotia
   5820 University Avenue
   Halifax, NS B3H 1V7
   (902) 428-4209

Ontario

Breast Cancer Information and
Education Services
   51 Hillcrest Avenue
   St. Catharines, ON L2R 4Y3
   (905) 687-3333

Burlington Breast Cancer Support
Service
   777 Guelph Line
   Burlington, ON L7R 3N2
   (416) 634-2333
   email: bbcss@wchat.on.ca

Canadian Cancer Society
   1639 Yonge Street
   Toronto, ON M4T 2W6
   (416) 488-5400

Cancer Information Service
   755 Concession Street
   Hamilton, ON L8V 1C4
   (905) 387-1153 or 1-800-263-6750
   Fax (905) 387-0376

Connecting Rainbows
   c/o 109 Booth Drive
   Stouffville, ON L4A 4S1
   (905) 642-2329

Helping You Helps Me
   244 Hugel Avenue
   Midland, ON L2R 1T2
   (705) 527-6278

Mind over Cancer
   53 Gillespie Crescent
   Ottawa, ON K1V 0W2
   (613) 738-1017

Ontario Breast Cancer Information
Exchange Pilot Project
   c/o Toronto-Bayview Regional Cancer
   Centre
   2075 Bayview Avenue
   Toronto, ON M4N 8M5
   (416) 480-5899
   Fax (416) 480-6002

Ontario Cancer Institute
   Princess Margaret Hospital
   500 Sherbourne Street
   Toronto, ON M4X 1K9
   (416) 924-0671

Thunder Bay Regional Cancer Centre
290 Munro Street
Thunder Bay, ON P7A 7T1
(807) 345-2030

Toronto-Bayview Sunnybrook Cancer
Centre
2075 Bayview Avenue
Toronto, ON M4N 3M5
(416) 4188-5801
Fax (416) 480-6220

Prince Edward Island

Atlantic Breast Cancer Information
Project
1 Rochford Street, Suite 1
Charlottetown, PEI C1A 3T1
(902) 892-9531
Fax (902) 628-8281

Canadian Cancer Society
P.O. Box 115
Charlottetown, PEI C1A 7K2
(902) 566-4007

Department of Health and Social
Services
Oncology Division
P.O. Box 2000
Charlottetown, PEI C1A 7P1
(902) 522-6027

Quebec

Breast Cancer Action
5890 Monkland, Suite 203
Montreal, QC H4A 1G2
(514) 483-1846
Fax (514) 482-1445

Canadian Cancer Society
5151, boulevard l'Assomption
Montreal, QC H1T 4A9
(514) 255-5151

Quebec Breast Cancer Information
Project
3840 rue Saint Urbain
Montreal, QC H2W 1T8
(514) 843-2930

Réseau d'échange l'information du
Québec sur le cancer du sein
c/o Hotel-Dieu de Montrél
3840 rue St.-Urbain
Pavillion de Bullion, bureau 6-108
Montréal, QC H2W1T8
(514) 843-2930
Fax (514) 843-2932

Tele Cancer/Infor Cancer
2075 Champlain Street
Montreal, PQ H2L 2T1
In Montreal: (514) 522-6237
Outside Montreal: 1-800-361-4212

Saskatchewan

Allan Blair Memorial Clinic
    4101 Dewdney Avenue
    Regina, SK S4T 7T1
    (306) 766-2333

Canadian Cancer Society
    201-2445 13th Avenue
    Regina, SK S4P 0W1
    (306) 757-4260

Saskatchewan Cancer Foundation
    2631 28th Avenue
    Regina, SK S4S 6X3
    (306) 5185-1831

BREAST CANCER ADVOCACY AND SUPPORT GROUPS

Note: Cities and phone numbers provided only.

INTERNATIONAL

Note: Canada is listed separately.

Australia

The Breast Cancer Support Service,
    Queensland; (07) 257-1155

New Zealand

Breast Cancer Support Society,
    affiliated with the Cancer Society of
    New Zealand, Auckland;
    (09) 524-0023

Federation of Women's Health Councils
    Aotearoa-New Zealand, Auckland;
    (09) 520-5175

Puerto Rico

Preventing and Surviving Breast Cancer
    Project, Taller Salud, Rio Piedras; (809)
    764-9639

United Kingdom

Breast Care & Mastectomy Association,
    London, England; helpline:
    (071) 867-1103; main number:
    (071) 867-8275; Glasgow, Scotland
    helpline (041) 353-1050

Women's Nationwide Cancer Control
    Campaign, London, England;
    helpline: (071) 729-2229;
    main number: (071) 729-4688

UNITED STATES
National

National Alliance of Breast Cancer
Organizations
    New York, NY
    (212) 719-0154

National Black Leadership Initiative on
Cancer
    Los Angeles, CA
    1-800-262-5429

National Breast Cancer Coalition,
    Washington, D.C.
    1-800-935-0434 or (202) 296-7477

Susan G. Komen Breast Cancer
Foundation
    Dallas, TX
    (214) 450-1777

Y-ME
    Homewood, IL
    National hotline 1-800-221-2141;
    24-hour hotline (708) 799-8228;
    Business number (708) 799-8338

Statewide
Alabama

Women to Woman, Gasden;
    (205) 543-8896

Alaska

Anchorage Women's Breast Cancer
    Support Group; (907) 261-3151

Arkansas

Phillips Cancer Support House,
    Fort Smith; (501) 782-6302

California

Bay Area Black Women's Health Project,
    Oakland; (510) 533-6923

Breast Cancer Action,
    San Francisco; (415) 922-8279

Women of Color Breast Cancer
Survivors Support Group,
    Los Angeles; (213) 294-7195

Women's Cancer Resource Center,
    Berkeley; (510) 548-9272,

Connecticut

Women Together, Danbury;
    (203) 790-9151 or (203) 790-6568

Delaware

Looking Ahead,
    Wilmington; (302) 652-LIFE

District of Columbia

Greater Washington Coalition for
    Cancer Survivorship; (202) 384-6422

Mary-Helen for Lesbians with Cancer;
    (202) 332-5536

Florida

Just Us, Miami; (305) 387-7549

Hawaii

Breast Cancer Support Group,
 Queen's Medical Center, Honolulu;
 (808) 537-7555

Idaho

Idaho Breast Cancer Coalition, Boise;
 Cordelia Persigehl; (208) 386-2764

Illinois

Cancer Support Network,
 Bloomington; (309) 828-9296

Kansas

Victory In the Valley, Wichita;
 (316) 262-4040 or 1-800-657-7202

Louisiana

Louisiana Breast Cancer Task Force,
 Harvey (New Orleans area);
 (504) 368-2493

Maine

The HOPE Group,
 South Paris; (207) 827-3753

Maryland

Advocacy Committee for Breast Cancer
 Survivors, Bethesda; (301) 718-7293

Massachusetts

Women's Community Cancer Project,
 Cambridge; (617) 354-9888

Valley's Women's Health Project
 (lesbians and their families);
 Amherst (413) 548-9431

Michigan

"EXPRESSIONS" for Women;
 East Grand Rapids (616) 957-3223

Missouri

Breast Cancer Network,
 Mid-America Cancer Center,
 Springfield; Brenda Monroe
 (417) 885-2565 or 1-800-432-CARE

New Jersey

Breast Cancer Resource Center,
 Princeton; (609) 497-2126

Montclair-North Essex YWCA
 Women's Center; (201) 746-5400

New Mexico

New Mexico Breast Cancer Coalition,
 Albuquerque; (505) 268-2899

New York

Brass Ears, Binghamton; (607) 648-3871

The Long Island 1 in 9 Breast Cancer
 Action Coalition; (516) 877-4370

SHARE,
 New York; (212) 719-4454 (Spanish);
 (718) 296-7108 (Chinese)

North Carolina

The Charlotte Organization for Breast
 Cancer Education; (704) 846-2190

Ohio

Cancer Family Care, Cincinnati;
 (513) 731-3346

Pennsylvania

Linda Creed Breast Cancer Foundation,
   Philadelphia; (215) 955-4354

Rhode Island

The HOPE Center for Life
   Enhancement, Providence;
   (401) 454-0404

South Dakota

Friends Against Breast Cancer,
   Sioux Falls; (605) 339-HELP

Native American Women's Health
   Education Resource Center,
   Lake Andes; (605) 487-7072

Tennessee

The Breast Concerns and Mastectomy
   Support Group, Nashville;
   (615) 665-0628

Texas

Rosebuds, Joan Gordon Center,
   Houston; (713) 665-2729 or
   (713) 668-2996

Vermont

Breast Cancer Action Group,
   Burlington; (802) 863-3507

Virginia

Virginia Breast Cancer Foundation,
   Richmond; (804) 740-3446

Wyoming

Support Group, Riverton, Nance Shelsta;
   (307) 858-7457

BREAST CANCER ONLINE

Through the Internet, you can participate in news groups and bulletin boards (public forums) on breast cancer. These can be accessed through either independent Internet providers or through an interactive computer service, such as CompuServe, Prodigy, or America Online (AOL).

Literature searches are great ways of getting specific information. Medline is the best search service for medical journal articles (many of which are extremely technical), and it also has a separate search service called Cancerlit. Compuserve, Prodigy, or America Online all give you access to Medline. Medline is also available through many public and university libraries all over North America.

Another way of accessing useful information is through a web browser, such as Netscape. By web browsing, you can go to various sites in cyberspace to find your information. When you don't know the worldwide web (www) address, use a search engine such as Yahoo or Webcrawler to search for what you want and simply type in your topic. The more specific you can be in your search, the better. For example, if you want information on mammography, don't type *breast cancer*, type *mammography*. A search engine is essentially an index to the Internet.

Once the search engine completes its search, a list of various sites will come up on your screen. These sites will range from promotional websites from, say, prosthesis stores, to university bulletin boards, to pepperings of articles. When you go to a site, you can save or print the information. Flashing text (called hypertext) is a sign that you'll get more information when you click on it. This may even link you to other sites on the Internet. A good resource is *Internet for Dummies*, which will walk you through Internet access step by step.

A FEW SITES TO GET YOU STARTED

alt.support.cancer
on-line discussion

cancernetaicicc.nci.nih.gov
National Cancer Institute

Gopher<\@>nih.gov
NCI's CancerNet

http://cancer.med.upenn.edu
The University of Pennsylvania's
    Oncolink

http://hpbl.nwc.ca/HealthNet

http://hyrax.med.uth.tmc.edu
The University of Texas on-line center for
    medical information

http://vh.radiology.ulowa.edu
The University of Iowa's "Virtual
    Hospital"

http://www.cancer.org.
American Cancer Society

http://www.gsa.gov/staff/pa/cic/html
Consumer Information Center

http://www.ihr.com
Internet Health Resources

http://www.nlm.nih.gov
National Library of Medicine

sci.med and sci.bio
on-line discussion
http://nysernet.org/breast/default.html
Breast Cancer Information
    Clearinghouse

http://wchat.on.ca/web/bbcss
Burlington Breast Cancer Support
    Services, Inc. (Burlington, Ontario,
    Canada)

INDEX

M. Sara Rosenthal is a professional health writer, teacher, and author of several books, including *The Gynecological Sourcebook, The Thyroid Sourcebook,* and *The Breastfeeding Sourcebook.* Her interest in health issues was triggered by her own experience with cancer at the age of twenty. An Associate of the Centre for Health Promotion at the University of Toronto (a World Health Organization collaborating center), Rosenthal is involved with lobbying for cancer prevention guidelines and lectures to organizations about health issues. She lives in Etobicoke, Canada.